Human Factors in Paramedic Practice
Second Edition

Edited by
Gary Rutherford

Disclaimer

Class Professional Publishing have made every effort to ensure that the information, tables, drawings and diagrams contained in this book are accurate at the time of publication. The book cannot always contain all the information necessary for determining appropriate care and cannot address all individual situations; therefore, individuals using the book must ensure they have the appropriate knowledge and skills to enable suitable interpretation. Class Professional Publishing does not guarantee, and accepts no legal liability of whatever nature arising from or connected to, the accuracy, reliability, currency or completeness of the content of *Human Factors in Paramedic Practice*. Users must always be aware that such innovations or alterations after the date of publication may not be incorporated in the content. Please note, however, that Class Professional Publishing assumes no responsibility whatsoever for the content of external resources in the text or accompanying online materials.

Text © Gary Rutherford 2022

All rights reserved. Without limiting the rights under copyright reserved above, no part of this publication may be reproduced, stored in or introduced into a retrieval system, or transmitted, in any form or by any means (electronic, mechanical, photocopying, recording or otherwise) without the prior written permission of the publisher of this book.

The information presented in this book is accurate and current to the best of the authors' knowledge.

The authors and publisher, however, make no guarantee as to, and assume no responsibility for, the correctness, sufficiency or completeness of such information or recommendation.

Printing history

First edition published 2020 (reprinted 2021)

Second edition published 2022

The authors and publisher welcome feedback from the users of this book. Please contact the publisher:

Class Professional Publishing,
The Exchange, Express Park, Bristol Road, Bridgwater TA6 4RR
Telephone: 01278 472 800
Email: post@class.co.uk
Website: www.classprofessional.co.uk

Class Professional Publishing is an imprint of Class Publishing Ltd

A CIP catalogue record for this book is available from the British Library

Paperback ISBN: 9781801610124

Cover design by Hybert Design Limited, UK

Designed and typeset by S4Carlisle Publishing Services

Printed in the UK by Short Run Press

This book is printed on paper from responsible sources. Refer to local recycling guidance on disposal of this book.

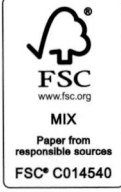

I would highly recommend this book, not only to paramedics but also to their colleagues in healthcare. It has been written by a premier league team of human factors specialists and frontline experts who share their knowledge and experience of applying human factors science to paramedic practice. It's very accessible, has a sound evidence base, and features many practical examples showing how to apply the tools and techniques.

Rhona Flin, Professor of Industrial Psychology, Robert Gordon University

We are entering an era where healthcare will be truly seen as a safety critical industry. The nature of paramedic practice in particular will need a well-informed professional workforce who are able to examine the systems and conditions they work in to understand how to make the care they provide as safe and effective as possible. This book will be essential reading for paramedics in all practice settings as it covers the key elements which will allow paramedics to better understand the complex sociotechnical realities of the care they provide to patients.

Andy Collen, author of *Decision Making in Paramedic Practice*

Contents

About the Authors vii
Acknowledgements xi
Forewords xii
Preface xv

1: **Introduction to Human Factors** 1
  Gary Rutherford

2: **Human Factors and Ergonomics: Past and Present** 15
  Steven Shorrock

3: **'Human Error'** 23
  Gary Rutherford

4: **Systems Thinking** 31
  Duncan McNab and Gary Rutherford

5: **Human-Centred Design** 49
  Shelly Jeffcott

6: **The Patient: An Element of the System** 71
  Gary Rutherford and Michael Moneypenny

7: **Well-Being of the Paramedic** 83
  Jo Mildenhall

8: **Situation Awareness and Decision Making** 101
  Ben Shippey and Gary Rutherford

9: **Teamwork in Paramedic Practice** 125
  Mike Christian and Neil Jeffers

Contents

10: Learning from Events — 141
Paul Bowie and Gary Rutherford

11: Safety Culture: Theory and Practice — 157
Steven Shorrock and Paul Bowie

Index — 171

About the Authors

Editor

Gary Rutherford is the Patient Safety Lead for the Scottish Ambulance Service. He is a paramedic and his interest in human factors originated from crew resource management training and application as a helicopter paramedic in Glasgow. Gary moved into paramedic education and was the programme lead for the DipHE in Paramedic Practice programme in Scotland. In this role, he designed and delivered a university module on human factors in paramedic practice. He is also an honorary educational co-ordinator at the Scottish Centre for Simulation and Clinical Human Factors. He has completed a BSc in Paramedic Practice, gained the Diploma in Immediate Medical Care awarded by the Royal College of Surgeons of Edinburgh, and completed postgraduate certificates in Learning and Teaching in Higher Education, and Patient Safety and Clinical Human Factors.

Contributors

Paul Bowie is a safety scientist, medical educator and chartered ergonomist and human factors specialist with NHS Education for Scotland based in Glasgow, where he is Programme Director (Safety and Improvement) and Director of the Safety, Skills and Improvement Research Collaborative. He has worked in the NHS in Scotland for over 25 years in a range of quality and safety advisory roles. He gained his doctorate in significant event analysis from the University of Glasgow in 2004 and has published over 120 articles in international peer-reviewed journals and co-edited a book on safety and improvement in healthcare. Paul is also Honorary Professor and a PhD supervisor/examiner at the University of Glasgow. He is an Honorary Fellow of the Royal College of Physicians of Edinburgh and the Royal College of General Practitioners, and a Registered Member of the Chartered Institute of Ergonomics and Human Factors.

Mike Christian is a consultant physician from Canada and a senior healthcare sector leader with nearly 30 years of experience, beginning as a paramedic. His specialties include critical care medicine, infectious diseases, military, aviation and pre-hospital medicine. Mike has enjoyed a diverse range of roles, including Chief Safety Officer for the largest multi-site hospital in Ontario, Canada, Medical Director of Critical Care Response Teams in Canada, and Director (Founding Board) of Ontario Agency for Health Protection and Promotion. In 2016, Mike moved to the UK for a sabbatical with London's Air Ambulance. He served as Clinical Lead for an air ambulance in the counties and subsequently was recruited to join London's Air Ambulance's senior team to lead on the delivery of key objectives within their research strategy. Mike completed an MSc in Public Health at the London

About the Authors

School of Hygiene and Tropical Medicine. He is a retired member of the Regular Forces of the RCAF and continues to serve as a reserve specialist medical officer/flight surgeon.

Shelly Jeffcott has academic qualifications in psychology, computing science and engineering design. She has worked as an applied human factors and ergonomics (HF/E) specialist embedded within healthcare teams in Australia and the UK for over 15 years. Shelly moved from her native Australia to Scotland in 2012 and has been working to integrate HF/E into local and national capability building programmes across NHS Scotland, via her roles at Healthcare Improvement Scotland, NHS Lothian, NHS Education for Scotland and the Scottish Ambulance Service. Shelly is passionate about HF/E and using design to improve quality and safety. Crucially this should incorporate those at the frontline, both delivering and receiving care. She is keen to support improvement work that uses systems approaches to deal with complexity and which considers the nature and context of care delivery, in terms of the way that work is done and not just as imagined.

Neil Jeffers spent seven years in the Territorial Army where he undertook a patrol medics course and developed his interest in medicine. Since he started flying helicopters 22 years ago, Neil has been Chief Pilot and Chief Flight Instructor for two companies and held instructor and examiner ratings on seven different types of helicopter. For the last 12 years, Neil has been flying at London's Air Ambulance and has been the Chief Pilot for the last five years. Neil has also spent the last ten years researching and teaching Human Factors and Team Resource Management to clinicians, lecturing at the International Masters (MSc) in Pre-hospital Critical Care at the University of Stavanger, Norway, The Institute of Pre-hospital Care and the Paramedic Science course at the University of Hertfordshire. Neil completed 14 desert marathons to raise money for London's Air Ambulance including the infamous Marathon des Sables.

Duncan McNab is a partner in a GP practice and an Assistant GP Director at NHS Education for Scotland. This role involves working nationally to develop, deliver and evaluate training and resources for frontline health and care teams in Quality Improvement and patient safety. Previously, Duncan worked as the clinical lead for patient safety in primary care in Ayrshire and Arran. Through these roles he developed an interest in human factors, especially in how work in complex systems can be optimised. He is currently working towards a PhD at the University of Glasgow applying a resilience engineering approach to explore how safety is created within primary care interdisciplinary work systems.

Jo Mildenhall is Clinical Lead for Mental Health at South Western Ambulance Service NHS Foundation Trust. Prior to this, she had over 20 years' frontline operational experience as a paramedic, mentor and team leader. Following her attendance at a rail crash early in her career, Jo developed an interest in staff psychological welfare and the impact of distress within emergency organisations. Jo graduated with an MA in Trauma Psychology and is undertaking a PhD, researching this area further. Jo was awarded a Winston Churchill Memorial Trust international research fellowship in

2019, travelling to Australia and New Zealand to study practical mental health and well-being strategies for paramedics. She also sits as a member on the College of Paramedics' Paramedic Mental Health and Wellbeing specialist interest group and contributes to the Royal College of Surgeons of Edinburgh's psychosocial and mental healthcare guidance for pre-hospital care practitioners and emergency responders.

Michael Moneypenny has degrees in Biochemistry and Medicine, and an MD in Medical Education. He is a consultant in anaesthesia and faculty member of the Scottish Centre for Simulation and Clinical Human Factors. His interests include the power gradients in healthcare, systems approaches to patient safety and the most effective methods for delivering simulation-based medical education. Dr Moneypenny is also President-Elect of the Association for Simulated Practice in Healthcare.

Ben Shippey is a Consultant Intensivist in NHS Tayside, having trained in the Midlands, East Anglia and South East Scotland. He has been involved in simulation-based medical education throughout his career, and is Educational Co-ordinator at the Scottish Centre for Simulation and Clinical Human Factors. He has developed and continues to deliver educational interventions with a non-technical skills theme to undergraduate and postgraduate healthcare professionals, and is advising the Royal College of Anaesthetists with regard to its future curriculum development in this domain. Ben has been involved in the organisation of pre-hospital care for motorsports events for the last 25 years, from club level to international events including the British Grand Prix, World Endurance Championship and British Touring Car Championship. He is Chief Medical Officer for the British round of the World Rally Championship.

Steven Shorrock is a Chartered Psychologist and Chartered Ergonomist and Human Factors Specialist with experience in aviation, rail, onshore process industries, healthcare and government administration. He has a BSc (Hons) in Applied Psychology, an MSc (Eng) in Work Design and Ergonomics, and a PhD on human error analysis and prediction. Since 1997, he has worked in industry and academia on projects spanning several European countries. He has developed a range of human factors tools used internationally and co-written a number of white papers (EUROCONTROL/FAA/UK CAA). He works at EUROCONTROL as a senior safety and human factors specialist, and is Editor-in-Chief of *HindSight* magazine. He was an invited member of the ICAO (International Civil Aviation Organization) Human Performance Task Force and Adjunct Associate Professor at the University of the Sunshine Coast. He blogs at https://humanisticsystems.com and co-edited *Human Factors and Ergonomics in Practice: Improving performance and well-being in the real world* (CRC Press).

Acknowledgements

I would like to thank all the contributors for their enthusiasm to share their knowledge and experience in order to enhance pre-hospital care, and for the support and encouragement they have given me during the process. Thanks also to Karen Hamilton, Owen Williams, Charlie Till, Scott MacKenzie, Scott Diamond, Andy Collen and Drew Inglis for reviewing earlier drafts of various chapters, and to Lianne Sherlock, senior editor at Class Professional Publishing for guidance and support throughout.

Foreword

The College of Paramedics is delighted to partner with Class Publishing on a range of textbooks for aspiring, newly qualified and advanced paramedics. The vision of the College is to inspire and enable all paramedics to participate in the profession within an environment based on safety, collegiality, inclusiveness, mental and physical wellbeing and innovation.
Paramedicine has developed exponentially in recent years. As a profession we are increasingly more involved in an ever-widening spectrum of healthcare.

Our textbooks, published by Class Publishing, will help you to take an evidence-based approach to your practice, as you develop your career. It would not be an exaggeration to say that Class Publishing's books and apps have made a true and lasting impact on the UK ambulance service and wider prehospital care arena.

Tracy Nicholls, Chief Executive, College of Paramedics

Foreword

On 29th March 2005, human factors touched my life in a way that I never expected, and in a way that I can never forget.

Elaine, mum to our two young children, was about to undergo a routine procedure. She was being cared for by a very experienced team in well-equipped surroundings. With the value of hindsight, if you had to list the clinical skills her team would need that day, you would have found those skills in abundance. If you'd listed all the equipment the team might need, you would have found it there that day. But that day was Elaine's last conscious one on Earth.

The emergency that interrupted the attempt to anaesthetise Elaine was unforeseeable. But the response was a disaster. The team lost situational awareness; decision making became fixated; leadership unclear and unco-ordinated; priorities confused. Attempts to use equipment were complicated by unfamiliarity. Within the team, some had the capacity to recover the situation safely but their attempts to communicate were ineffectual and stifled. This was caused partly by behaviours on that day, but mostly by the culture created long before that day.

The issue wasn't their technical skills; it was their non-technical skills. This wasn't about having the right equipment and processes; this was about having equipment and processes that made it easy to get it right. This wasn't about the culture of their organisation; it was about the culture across healthcare in 2005.

As an airline pilot, I'm familiar with human factors; I've been taught and examined on it as a theoretical topic. But I've learned much more about human factors and systems thinking every day of my job. I see the impact of good design; I see the impact of good non-technical skills; I see the impact of a just and safe culture. The steady and remarkable improvement in safety in aviation over decades has, to a significant extent, been driven by the science of Human Factors. Yet at first in healthcare, I witnessed a lack of desire to adopt a systems thinking approach to understand how all of these workplace elements had interacted on the day. All I wanted was for this not to happen to someone else.

The good news is that healthcare is slowly waking up to human factors and systems thinking, but even in the best designed system the human remains the final line of defence. That's you. Your technical knowledge remains the foundation and with human factors science, the application of this foundation will be easier and more effective. And will *usually* – a word I don't use lightly – be the reason for success or failure.

Foreword

After Elaine's death, as I started to re-build my life, I began working with some amazing healthcare people and human factors professionals. I simply wanted to promote an understanding of the science. This book does that in a way that I wish I had done. Perhaps it's not surprising that many of the experts I look up to have contributed. And it's perhaps even less surprising that the editor is a paramedic because it has been those who are involved in applying skills in moments where time is in short supply that have embraced human factors thinking the most.

If I have one criticism of this masterful piece of work: it is aimed at one group in healthcare. This book is too good for one profession. This book needs to be read by those in all safety-critical industries.

Martin Bromiley OBE FRCSEd (ad hom)
Founder, Clinical Human Factors Group
Airline Training Captain and Crew Resource Management Trainer
23rd of May 2020

Preface

I was first introduced to 'human factors' during the Crew Resource Management (CRM) sessions of my HEMS crewmember course in 2006, prior to commencing a 6-year period as an air ambulance paramedic with Helimed 5 in Glasgow. Like many other paramedics who have completed this type of non-technical skills training, I thoroughly enjoyed the topic. I think this was because it was new to me and different from the clinical and technical skills learning that had been the focus of my development up to that point. I'm sure that I was also intrigued, as are most people, about instances when things go wrong or people make mistakes. The CRM training incorporated films and case studies of aviation-related incidents to powerfully illustrate the importance of non-technical skills such as situation awareness, decision making, communication, teamwork and leadership. I can recall that these sessions focused my mind on how I could contribute to safe flight operations. Annual CRM theory update sessions were held, although the challenge was applying the theory to practice. The pilots obviously had much more experience in practical application, and I can remember many flights, incidents and debriefs with them, where both good and suboptimal non-technical skills were evident.

In 2010, I heard airline captain Martin Bromiley OBE give a presentation at the Emergency Medical Retrieval Service conference, where he spoke about the death of his wife Elaine during 'a routine operation'. Martin delivered a very powerful talk, which had a profound effect on myself and others in the audience. It created a bit of a 'lightbulb moment' for me, as Martin outlined how the CRM branch of 'human factors' that is practised by airline crews also had potential for application in healthcare to benefit patient safety.

My interest and understanding related to 'human factors' has continued since, and more recently I have grown to appreciate that it is much broader than just the CRM/non-technical skills training application. 'Human factors' as an approach to system improvement is gaining momentum in healthcare, with increasing literature and communities of practice emerging. Through these, it is becoming clearer that it is a distinct discipline that looks to understand the wider work system interactions and performance when things go well and don't go so well. It then uses this understanding to design or strengthen the system to achieve benefits.

This book is intended to be an introduction to the discipline of 'human factors', highlighting some of its main principles and relating them to aspects of paramedic practice. The main aims are to consider the various definitions and perceptions of the concept of 'human factors', and to bring the systems thinking and design aspects forward, while also acknowledging some of the cognitive psychology and human-to-human interaction elements that form the basis of CRM principles. The intent of

Preface

the book is to constructively challenge some of the current understanding of 'human factors' in healthcare and encourage healthy conversations for its development and application in paramedic practice. There are many situations in pre-hospital care and paramedic practice where 'human factors' approaches can be applied, therefore the examples given in this book are not the only ones relevant. The challenge to you as you gain more of an understanding of the key principles of 'human factors' is to try to look for instances where they can be applied in your practice.

The contributors to the book are all experts in their field with specialism or practical experience in the application of 'human factors' approaches, and all have experience in pre-hospital care, or working with ambulance services or the wider health service. I would be keen to state that I do not consider myself a 'human factors' specialist, and the purpose of this book is not to turn you into one, but I am an advocate for its concepts and would like to encourage others to consider how 'human factors' can be applied to promote improved patient safety within healthcare.

I have thoroughly enjoyed reading and learning more about the discipline from the contributors' chapters. I'm certain that my journey (and that of healthcare) in understanding 'human factors' is far from complete, and I hope that this book contributes to future developments and stimulates further discussion in the years ahead. I also hope that you enjoy the book and find it helpful as you apply these concepts to your role as a healthcare professional and forge ahead with your own journey of understanding 'human factors'.

Gary Rutherford
May 2020

Terminology

Please note that we have used the terms 'paramedic' and 'ambulance clinician' interchangeably, in an effort to vary the language and also consider a range of readers. It is not intended to indicate that some aspects are applicable to paramedics and others to technicians, students, learners or support workers. The same should be considered with the terms 'pre-hospital care' and 'ambulance services'. Many of the principles will be applicable to pre-hospital care providers and organisations that are not ambulance services.

Chapter 1
Introduction to Human Factors

Gary Rutherford

> In this chapter:
> - An introduction to the principles and aims of human factors
> - Consideration of definitions, terminology and models related to human factors
> - How human factors can influence patient safety

Introduction

'Human factors' is a term that most pre-hospital providers will have heard of, as it is being increasingly referred to in healthcare. Since the 1940s, human factors principles and specialists have become embedded in a range of high reliability and safety-critical industries such as mining, oil and gas extraction, construction, military, aviation, rail and nuclear power generation. Healthcare has noticed the benefits achieved by these industries in improving reliability and safety, and has therefore been exploring and evaluating ways to implement human factors principles. Healthcare is in the infancy of its understanding and application of human factors, and the same can be said specifically for the pre-hospital world that we are interested in. There are a few challenges associated with applying human factors approaches, including gaining a shared understanding of what it is. Therefore, this book offers an introduction to the topic of human factors, outlining some of the key principles and how they can be considered and applied in paramedic practice.

What is Human Factors?

Today's understanding of human factors has its origins in military aviation from around the time of World War II, which is discussed further in Chapter 2. Since then, the concept has grown and been applied in many other high-risk industries. Human factors is described as 'a science at the intersection of psychology and engineering' (Russ et al, 2013), which encourages a systems approach to consider a range of aspects related to human work. These aspects include how humans interact with each other and with other elements of the system, for example, the tools, technology, processes and tasks that are required to do the work. It is an approach that takes

Chapter 1 – Introduction to Human Factors

account of the capabilities and limitations of humans, in addition to cognitive, physical and organisational factors within the workplace (International Ergonomics Association, 2020). It uses this understanding of human performance in different circumstances to design the work environments, procedures, tasks and equipment to make it easy for people to use and interact with, instead of people having to adapt to poor design. Human factors therefore aims to improve the 'fit' between people and their environment to achieve a safer, more productive and effective workplace. In the first instance it would look to design the work system to fit the human, only attempting to make the human fit the work (through selection or training) when the first approach is not possible (Dul et al, 2012).

The International Ergonomics Association (IEA) proposes two interrelated aims of human factors:

- improve system performance (for example, safety, efficiency and productivity)
- optimise human well-being (for example, health and safety, experience and satisfaction).

The linked relationship between these aims is crucial and is illustrated in Figure 1.1. If system performance is improved, a benefit in human (staff and patient) well-being can be achieved. Equally, if well-being is optimised, positive results will be seen in overall system performance.

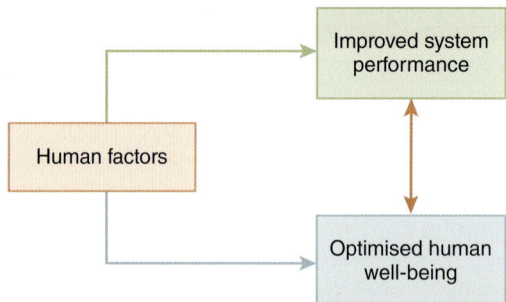

Figure 1.1 – Twin aims of human factors

In healthcare there are a range of views and thoughts on what human factors is. This is partly due to the breadth of the discipline and also the development that is taking place in relation to healthcare professionals' understanding of the subject. You may find the heading of this section odd – 'what *is* human factors?', not 'what *are* human factors?'. To use 'is' makes it clearer that we are predominantly considering human factors as a recognised discipline with defined principles and approaches to cover all of the above aspects. The use of 'are' to describe human factors may encourage the belief that it is an approach only related to factors associated with human behaviour. In response to this developing shared understanding, human factors is increasingly being recognised as a potential way of adding value to existing programmes and initiatives in healthcare, although it is principally being used at the moment to assist with reducing avoidable harm.

Definitions

Various definitions of human factors have been proposed, although the IEA offers the following definition which is a commonly cited description that can be applied across a range of industries:

> Ergonomics (or human factors) is the **scientific discipline** concerned with the understanding of **interactions among humans** and other **elements of a system**, and **the profession** that applies theory, principles, data and methods **to design** in order to **optimise human well-being** and overall **system performance**.
>
> (IEA, 2020)

As this is a rather lengthy definition with several elements and points, it can be helpful if we break it down to consider further (see Table 1.1).

Alternative Definitions

The Clinical Human Factors Group (CHFG) offers a definition that also highlights the design for the human work aspect of the discipline, while specifically considering the limitations and characteristics of people. They also introduce the concept of the socio-technical system, a term which captures the complexity of modern healthcare delivery.

> Human Factors (also called ergonomics) is a discipline that considers both the physical and mental characteristics of people as well as the organisational factors or wider socio-technical system. It is the application of scientific methods to the design and evaluation of tasks, jobs, equipment, environments and systems to make them more compatible with the needs, capabilities and limitations of people.
>
> (Clinical Human Factors Group, 2020)

These definitions attempt to cover all the main aspects, aims and outcomes of human factors, hence their intricacy. However, it may be helpfully captured well with this simple, concise definition:

> Understanding the interactions between people and all other elements within a system, and design in light of this understanding.
>
> (Wilson, 2014)

Socio-technical system – synergistic combination of humans, machines, environments, work activities and organisational structures and processes (Carayon et al, 2015).

Chapter 1 – Introduction to Human Factors

Table 1.1 – Breakdown of IEA definition of human factors/ergonomics

IEA Definition Key Point	Interpretation
Scientific discipline	An organised theoretical knowledge of a particular topic or a field of study.
Interactions among humans	Can include the interactions between healthcare staff and patients, and between healthcare staff in the workplace. Non-technical skills such as communication, teamwork and decision making can play an important role in these interactions.
Interactions among ... other elements of a system	A system is an interconnected network of elements that function together to produce an outcome or product. The other elements (in addition to the humans) are the tools and equipment, the tasks, the physical, social and cultural environments, and organisational policies and procedures influencing work.
The profession that applies ...	Human factors is also a recognised regulated profession with many registered human factors experts applying the principles in safety-critical industries (although not many in healthcare).
To design	This is one of the key points. It is fundamental that any understanding gained from the analysis of system interactions is used to design or strengthen the system to achieve improvements.
Optimise human well-being	One of the 'twin aims'. An understanding that optimal design of work systems can lead to staff feeling safe, supported and valued at work with increased job satisfaction and enjoyment. In the context of healthcare, the well-being of the patient can also be considered.
Overall system performance	The second 'twin aim'. If human factors principles can be applied to the design of workplace tasks and processes, the other outcome will be improved overall system performance. In healthcare, this could lead to safer care and better outcomes for patients.

Terminology

In these definitions you will see that 'ergonomics' is stated as an alternative term for human factors, and as you read more widely on this topic you will find that the terms human factors and ergonomics are both used in literature and practice. The Chartered Institute of Ergonomics and Human Factors (CIEHF) explains that, as the discipline evolved from the 1940s, some variation of terminology occurred in different countries. The CIEHF states that the terms human factors and ergonomics are viewed as the same discipline by the profession, therefore are synonymous and can be used interchangeably. They do acknowledge that ergonomics is often considered to be more related to the physical aspects of the workplace environment and human factors associated to the wider work system. Paramedics may be familiar with ergonomics in the context of moving and handling principles and techniques. While moving and handling is an element of the physical aspects of human work, it won't be addressed in this book, as other core texts are available on the topic. Both terms are acknowledged in the names of the CIEHF professional body in the UK and the Human Factors and Ergonomics Society in the USA. Therefore, to acknowledge the breadth of the discipline, the historical and geographical evolution, and synonymous use of 'human factors' and 'ergonomics', the abbreviation HF/E will be used throughout the book.

There are a couple of other terms that are closely associated with HF/E as understood by many in healthcare, and these will be discussed in other chapters of the book but are worth clarifying at this point:

Non-Technical Skills

Non-technical skills are 'the cognitive, social and personal skills that complement technical skills, and contribute to safe and effective task performance' (Flin et al, 2008). Non-technical skills such as situation awareness, decision making and teamwork, and how they can be affected by stress, design and unforeseen interactions, will be discussed later in the book. Although they are an important part of HF/E related to how individuals behave, interact and perform in teams, non-technical skills represent only a small proportion of the theory, practice and benefits of HF/E.

Crew Resource Management

Originally called Cockpit Resource Management (CRM), this concept originates from the aviation industry and is a team training approach that focuses on non-technical skills. The Civil Aviation Authority (CAA, 2016) describes how recordings from cockpit voice recorders (also known as black boxes) suggested that aviation incidents were related to failures of interpersonal skills, communication, decision making and leadership. CRM training was introduced in the 1980s to increase awareness and application of these non-technical skills to enhance flight safety. This was later extended to include other members of the flight crew, cabin crew, engineers and air traffic controllers and renamed Crew Resource Management. Team Resource Management (TRM) has the same team training and non-technical skills principles as CRM, although is generally applied in non-aviation environments. Therefore, CRM and HF/E are not the same thing, although it would be appropriate to consider CRM as a subcategory of HF/E that focuses on non-technical skills awareness, assessment and training.

Human Factors for Patient Safety

Patient safety is 'about maximising the things that go right and minimising the things that go wrong for people experiencing healthcare' (NHS Improvement, 2019), and is an essential element of providing a quality healthcare service. Modern healthcare

Chapter 1 – Introduction to Human Factors

provides many benefits in response to the investigation, diagnosis and treatment of a vast range of illnesses and injuries, to improve or maintain our health. However, on occasion, things can go wrong in healthcare leading to patients being harmed or exposed to potential harm. It is this actual or potential harm that has been the focus of most HF/E application in healthcare to date, although its application to helping ensure as many things as possible go right is starting to be recognised.

The concept of patient safety emerged just over 25 years ago (Vincent and Amalberti, 2016). During that period there have been several reports that have increased the understanding that patients in the healthcare system are exposed to avoidable harm. The publication of the Institute of Medicine (IoM) report 'To Err is Human: Building a Safer Health System' (2000) was a significant moment in the patient safety movement. Its headline statement was that between 44,000 and 98,000 people died each year in United States hospitals due to 'medical error', although this figure was extrapolated from four US hospitals. The Department of Health in the UK released their equivalent report in 2000, 'An Organisation with a Memory', which stated that around 10% of patients admitted to NHS hospitals experienced an adverse event that led to harm, with approximately 50% being considered avoidable. More recently, The Health Foundation (2011) reviewed research from the UK, Europe, USA and Australia to suggest that estimates of patient safety incident rates are variable, as is the strength of associated evidence. They report that:

- between 3% and 25% of patients admitted to hospital experience an adverse event
- one study of primary care patient records suggested that 9% contained an adverse event
- harm rates of 15% have been proposed in community hospitals.

Although the evidence regarding the incident rates of in-hospital patient safety events is variable, it has been noted that the evidence base and understanding related to pre-hospital patient safety and adverse event rates is even less established (Price et al, 2013; Fisher et al, 2015; Hagiwara et al, 2019). This may be due to a lack of focus on patient safety in pre-hospital care compared with acute hospital settings and the challenges of measuring patient safety in pre-hospital environments. After carrying out a retrospective review of ambulance service clinical records in Sweden, Hagiwara et al (2019) proposed a pre-hospital adverse event rate of 4.3%. Of these, 4% were classified as having potential for harm and 0.3% as actual harm identified. Much more research is required in this area to continue to build an

> *Patient safety incident – any unintended or unexpected incident which could have, or did, lead to harm for one or more patients receiving healthcare (NHS Improvement, 2017). It can also be referred to as an 'adverse event'.*

understanding of adverse event and harm rates in pre-hospital care. The IoM report goes on to state that when an adverse event occurs, seeking to apportion blame to individuals is a common reaction. 'Human error' or 'clinical error' (discussed further in Chapter 3) is often cited as the cause of an incident. However, it is increasingly recognised that when something goes wrong there are often multiple interacting contributory factors that combine to produce it, rather than it being caused by a single incorrect action of a worker. Professor Don Berwick, an expert in patient safety, was asked to lead a review of safety in NHS England after the publication of the Francis Report which investigated the care failings at Mid Staffordshire Hospitals between 2005 and 2009. In the Berwick report 'A Promise to Learn – A Commitment to Act' (Department of Health, 2013), the review group states:

- patient safety problems exist throughout healthcare
- healthcare staff are not to blame. The vast majority of healthcare staff come to work to do a good job and to be proud of their work
- good people can fail when working conditions do not provide the conditions for success
- a system devoted to continual learning and improvement is required
- blame and punishment should not be used for dealing with individuals who have made an error.

The concepts of human fallibility and adverse events can be viewed in one of two ways: a person-centred approach or a systems approach (Reason, 2000).

Person-Centred Approach

With this approach, the focus is on the performance of the individual clinicians involved in the patient safety incident. It may consider lack of attention, carelessness, or not 'applying the rules' as factors that directly 'cause' the issue. Understandably, this can lead to corrective action aimed at changing the unwanted human behaviour, for example, more training or guidance to be more vigilant, which may subsequently create a blame culture.

Systems Approach

A systems approach acknowledges that incidents and accidents will inevitably occur. Any 'errors' are viewed as a consequence or symptom of system design and interaction between elements in the system. When an adverse event occurs, the learning should be used to improve or re-design the systems to consider human abilities, limitations, needs and preferences to make it harder to do the wrong thing and easier to do the right thing.

This systems design approach is the foundation of the HF/E discipline. It can therefore be appreciated how the understanding and application of HF/E is key to enhancing patient safety.

Chapter 1 – Introduction to Human Factors

Safety-I and Safety-II

As we can see, the traditional view of patient safety since the 'To Err is Human' report has been to focus on when things go wrong. The existence of 'safety' has been considered to mean that 'as few things as possible go wrong'. Hollnagel et al (2015) define this view as 'Safety-I' and state that this approach waits for something to go wrong, then looks to identify and fix the 'causes' of the incident. However, highly complex and interacting systems, particularly those in the emergency setting, cannot be easily broken down to identify the problem (see Chapter 4). Therefore, an emerging belief is that safety should evolve from a view of 'as few things as possible go wrong' to consider how 'as many things as possible can go right'. This alternative view is referred to as Safety-II (Hollnagel et al, 2015). Safety-II considers the work processes and tasks when they are going well and suggests that this is not because humans are doing what they should, but because they adjust what they are doing to match the conditions. A Safety-II approach would seek to understand how things usually go right, and the role that humans play in adapting their performance and actions in order to meet variations in system demand. If the system operation can be understood when it is working well, it can be enhanced and strengthened to build in resilience for unexpected events.

Those that promote a Safety-II approach do not suggest that it should replace a Safety-I approach, but instead propose that a combination of both approaches may be the best way forward.

Misconceptions of HF/E

The challenges of defining HF/E and the lack of suitably qualified experts to guide understanding in healthcare may be reasons as to why it can be easy for misconceptions to become established. These misconceptions may slow the progress of HF/E development in healthcare (Russ et al, 2013). It could also be argued that the term 'human factors' is slightly misleading, as it may suggest a focus on factors only related to human performance and behaviour, i.e. the systems that we work in are perfectly safe, and problems only arise when humans are not careful or vigilant enough, make the wrong decisions or don't follow protocols. It is relatively common to hear problems that become apparent in healthcare described as 'caused by human factors', a view which fails to appreciate that HF/E science aims to design the system to improve performance. Therefore, 'human factors' should not be proposed as a cause or explanation for failure (Shorrock, 2019b).

Healthcare has also adopted the CRM team training principles from pilot training which focuses on the non-technical skills of the individual, rather than the wider principles of HF/E. This means that healthcare can often be of the incorrect opinion that CRM is the same as HF/E. This can be a prevalent view which has led to organisations believing that they have 'done human factors' after implementing training for staff in some aspects of non-technical skills. Russ et al (2013) 'separate fact from fiction' by proposing key concepts that are commonly misunderstood. They state that HF/E does not:

- look to eliminate 'human error'
- address problems by teaching people to modify their behaviour

- focus only on the individual
- consist of a limited set of principles that can be learnt during brief training.

Finally, the view that HF/E is just 'common sense' is also refuted (Shorrock, 2019a). When a task or interaction with equipment works well, it can often go unnoticed because it has been designed well. When this is reviewed with hindsight it can easily be mistaken as 'well that was just common sense to make it like that'. This dismisses the complexity of human work and the human-centred design approach (Chapter 5) that may have taken place. Common sense may be the view of those who confuse HF/E with 'behaving safely'.

Models for HF/E Application

Due to the breadth of the HF/E discipline, the range of theories that it draws from and the complexity and variation of workplaces, it can be challenging to present all of the key aspects in one model. Therefore, no single agreed model of HF/E exists. However, there are a number of models related to accident causation and system function that have developed and evolved, which can be helpful when applying HF/E approaches.

James Reason's 'Swiss Cheese' model is often associated with HF/E and may be one that you are familiar with. Reason (2008) describes that this model aims to illustrate 'how unsafe acts and latent conditions combine to breach the barriers and safeguards' within a complex system. Examples of latent conditions are organisational processes, management decisions, design of environments and cultures. The model is based on an analogy of slices of cheese, with each slice acting as a layer of defence within a system or organisation. Each slice has holes that are continually moving and changing size. However, the holes in each layer may align and allow the hazard to pass through the defences and cause an accident. Dekker (2014) acknowledges that barrier models like the 'Swiss Cheese' do generally turn people's attention 'upstream' to system factors, although he also suggests that they do not clearly illustrate *how* social, organisational and bureaucratic factors influence system defences.

Also, it is important to appreciate that it was intended to be used as a retrospective systemic accident model, therefore is more limited if used to try and make predictions before something has gone wrong, when everything in the system could potentially be identified as a latent condition. Reason (2008) also acknowledges that the linear structure, particularly of earlier versions of the 'Swiss Cheese' model, may lead to the search for elusive 'root causes' of an accident. The perceived limitations of this type of model have led to the development of other system models.

An 'onion' structure to illustrate how elements of systems interact with each other is a popular concept (Moray, 2000; World Health Organization, 2009; Wilson and Sharples, 2015). Although there are slight differences in the proposed layering and structure of these onion models, they are helpful to an extent in illustrating the various elements of socio-technical systems, i.e. where humans interact with each

Chapter 1 – Introduction to Human Factors

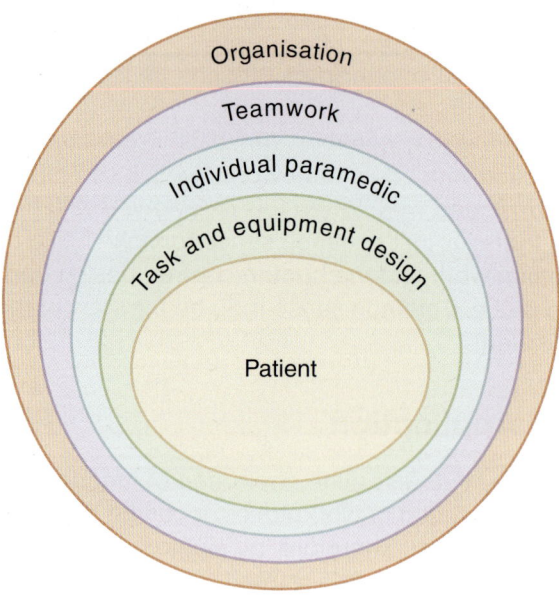

Figure 1.2 – HF/E 'onion'

other and the technical world in which they work. An example of an 'onion' model can be seen in Figure 1.2.

The Systems Engineering Initiative for Patient Safety (SEIPS) Model (Carayon et al, 2006) in Figure 1.3 expands further on these models and is specific to systems thinking and design for patient safety. It illustrates the 'work system' interactions in a more specific way than the 'Swiss Cheese' and 'onion' models. The SEIPS model also demonstrates how these interactions can lead to outcomes related to patients, employees and the organisation, which are aligned to the HF/E twin aims to improve well-being and system performance.

The SEIPS model was updated and extended in 2013 to SEIPS 2.0, although the original model has been chosen for this book as it is slightly easier to understand and has the same principles as the later version. Further discussion and application of the SEIPS model and also a framework for systems thinking, STEW (Systems Thinking for Everyday Work) is in Chapter 4.

Summary

HF/E is a scientific discipline which is used to understand human work, the interacting elements and design of a complex system, and to facilitate learning from events to improve system performance and human well-being. Many safety-critical industries apply and integrate HF/E principles to good effect and healthcare has started to adopt some of these concepts, although there is a lack of supporting policy attention in most modern healthcare systems. Although healthcare may largely have

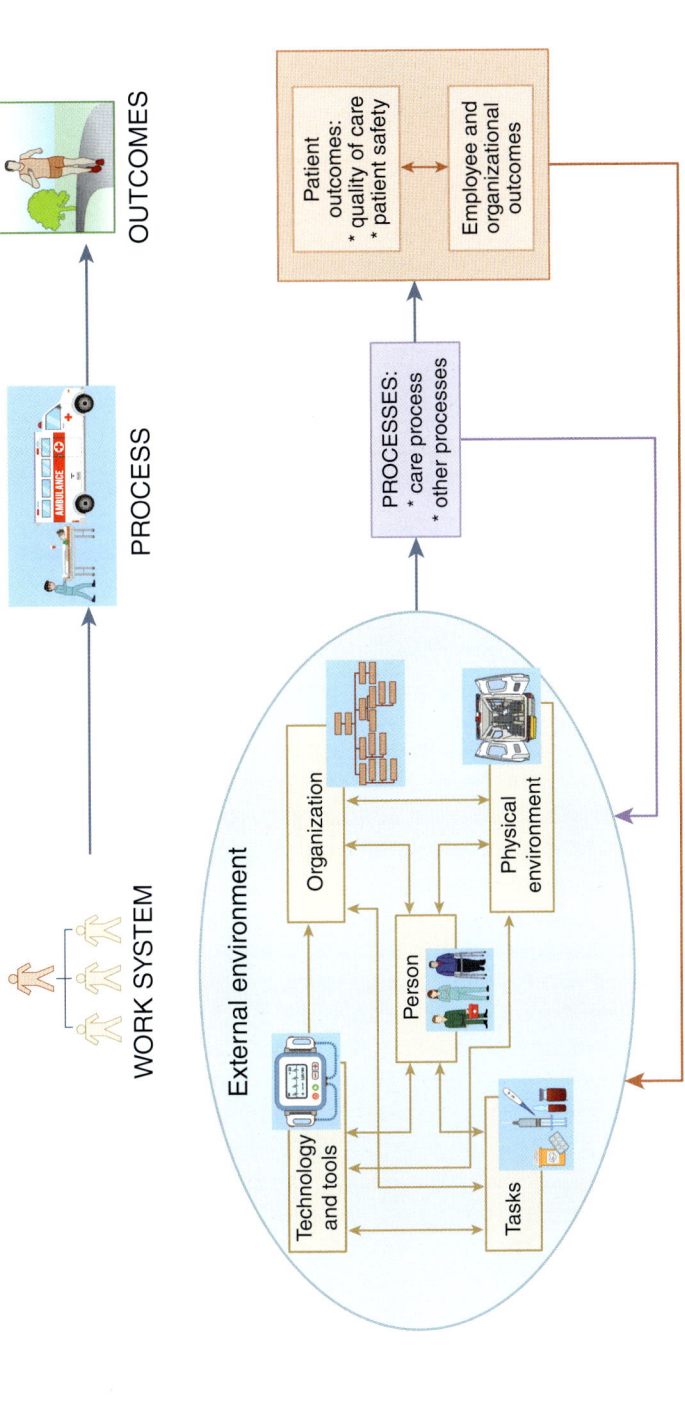

Figure 1.3 – Systems Engineering Initiative for Patient Safety

Source: Reproduced from Work system design for patient safety: the SEIPS model, Carayon et al, 15(Suppl 1), i51, 2006 with permission from BMJ Publishing Group Ltd.

Chapter 1 – Introduction to Human Factors

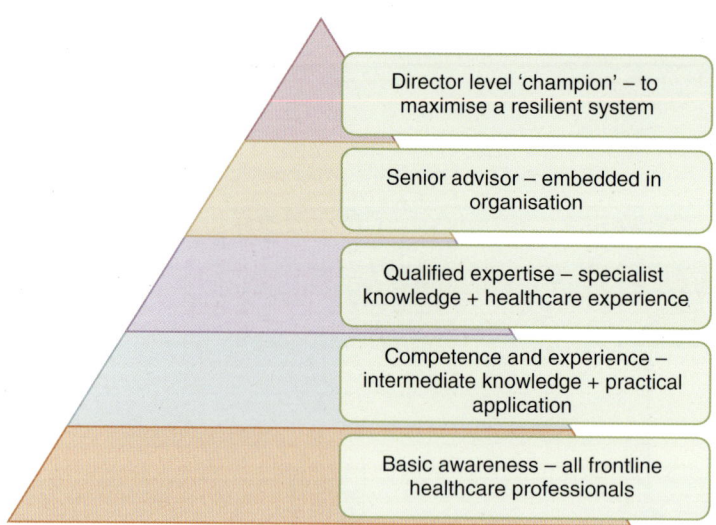

Figure 1.4 – Suggested levels of HF/E input in healthcare
Source: Chartered Institute of Ergonomics and Human Factors (2018). Adapted with permission

historically focused on non-technical skills, person-centred approaches and Safety-I views, it is now appreciating the benefits of the design-driven foundation and systems thinking approach of HF/E.

Patient safety as a concept continues to develop and evidence related to adverse events in pre-hospital care is immature. However, links between systems thinking and patient safety continue to become established across healthcare. Ambulance clinicians, pre-hospital care organisations and ultimately patients and service users will benefit if HF/E principles are adopted.

This book brings together subject matter experts to present an introduction to some of the key elements of HF/E, i.e. its history, systems thinking, human-centred design, interaction with the patient, non-technical skills of individuals and in teams, well-being, learning from events and safety culture. The purpose of the book is not to turn you into an HF/E 'expert'. The CIEHF proposes a pyramid structure to illustrate suggested levels of expertise that is required in healthcare organisations and professions (see Figure 1.4). They suggest that HF/E 'awareness' already exists across a range of healthcare professionals. The aims of the book are to increase ambulance staff awareness and competence levels related to HF/E, and to encourage pre-hospital care organisations to recognise when it would be beneficial to seek advice and expertise from suitably qualified HF/E experts.

References

Carayon, P. et al. (2006). Work system design for patient safety: the SEIPS model. *Quality & Safety in Health Care*. 15(Suppl 1): i50–i58.

Carayon, P. et al. (2015). Advancing a sociotechnical systems approach to workplace safety – developing the conceptual framework. *Ergonomics*. 58(4): 548–564.

Chartered Institute of Ergonomics and Human Factors (2018). Human Factors for Health & Social Care (White Paper) [online]. Available from: https://www.ergonomics.org.uk/Public/Resources/Publications/Healthcare-White-Paper/Public/Resources/Publications/Healthcare_White_Paper.aspx?hkey=caf8ec2c-9ad9-4335-952e-c01abcd5bfd1

Civil Aviation Authority (2016). Flight-crew human factors handbook: CAP737 [online]. West Sussex: Civil Aviation Authority. Available from: https://publicapps.caa.co.uk/docs/33/CAP%20737%20DEC16.pdf

Clinical Human Factors Group (2020). What are clinical human factors? [online]. https://chfg.org/what-are-clinical-human-factors/.

Dekker, S. (2014). *The Field Guide to Understanding 'Human Error'*. 3rd ed. Boca Raton: CRC Press.

Department of Health (2000). An organisation with a memory [online]. London: The Stationery Office. Available from: https://webarchive.nationalarchives.gov.uk/20130105144251/http://www.dh.gov.uk/prod_consum_dh/groups/dh_digitalassets/@dh/@en/documents/digitalasset/dh_4065086.pdf

Department of Health (2013). A promise to learn – a commitment to act [online]. London: Williams Lea. Available from: https://assets.publishing.service.gov.uk/government/uploads/system/uploads/attachment_data/file/226703/Berwick_Report.pdf

Dul, J. et al. (2012). A strategy for human factors/ergonomics: developing the discipline and profession. *Ergonomics*. 55(4): 377–395.

Fisher, J.D. et al. (2015). Patient safety in ambulance services: a scoping review. *Health Services and Delivery Research* [online]. 3(21). Available from: https://www.ncbi.nlm.nih.gov/pubmed/25996021

Flin, R., O'Connor, P., Crichton, M. (2008). *Safety at the Sharp End: A Guide to Non-Technical Skills*. Aldershot: Ashgate.

Hagiwara, M.A. et al. (2019). Adverse events in prehospital emergency care: a trigger tool study. *BMC Emergency Medicine*. 19: 14.

Healthcare Improvement Scotland (2018). Learning from adverse events through reporting and review – A national framework from Scotland [online]. Available from: http://www.healthcareimprovementscotland.org/our_work/governance_and_assurance/management_of_adverse_events/national_framework.aspx

Hollnagel, E., Wears, R.L., Braithwaite, J. (2015). From Safety-I to Safety-II: A White Paper [online]. Available from: https://www.england.nhs.uk/signuptosafety/wp-content/uploads/sites/16/2015/10/safety-1-safety-2-whte-papr.pdf

Institute of Medicine (2000). To Err is Human: Building a Safer Health System [online]. Washington, D.C.: National Academies Press. Available from: https://pubmed.ncbi.nlm.nih.gov/25077248/

International Ergonomics Association (2020). Human Factors/Ergonomics (HF/E): Definition and applications [online]. Available from: https://iea.cc/what-is-ergonomics/

Moray, N. (2000). Culture, politics and ergonomics. *Ergonomics*. 43(7): 858–868.

Chapter 1 – Introduction to Human Factors

NHS Improvement (2017). Report a patient safety incident [online]. Available from: https://improvement.nhs.uk/resources/report-patient-safety-incident/.

NHS Improvement & NHS England (2019). The NHS Patient Safety Strategy [online]. Available from: https://improvement.nhs.uk/documents/5472/190708_Patient_Safety_Strategy_for_website_v4.pdf

Price, R. et al. (2013). What causes adverse events in prehospital care? A human-factors approach. *Emergency Medical Journal*. 30: 583–588.

Reason, J. (2000). Human error: models and management. *British Medical Journal*. 320: 768–770.

Reason, J. (2008). *The Human Contribution: Unsafe acts, accidents and heroic recoveries*. Farnham: Ashgate.

Russ, A.L. et al. (2013). The science of human factors: separating fact from fiction. *BMJ Quality & Safety*. 22(10): 802–808.

Shorrock, S. (2019a). What Human Factors isn't: 1. Common Sense. *Humanistic Systems* [online]. Available from: https://humanisticsystems.com/

Shorrock, S. (2019b). What Human Factors isn't: 4. A Cause of Accidents. *Humanistic Systems* [online]. Available from: https://humanisticsystems.com/

The Health Foundation (2011). Evidence scan: Levels of harm [online]. Available from: https://www.health.org.uk/sites/default/files/LevelsOfHarm_0.pdf

Vincent, C., Amalberti, R. (2016). *Safer Healthcare: Strategies for the Real World*. London: Springer Open.

Wilson, J.R. (2014). Fundamentals of systems ergonomics/human factors. *Applied Ergonomics* [online]. 45(1): 5–13. Available from: https://www.ncbi.nlm.nih.gov/pubmed/23684119

Wilson, J.R., Sharples, S. (2015). *Evaluation of Human Work*. 4th Ed. Boca Raton: CRC Press.

World Health Organization (2009). Human Factors in Patient Safety: Review of Topics and Tools [online]. Available from: https://www.who.int/patientsafety/research/methods_measures/human_factors/human_factors_review.pdf

Chapter 2
Human Factors and Ergonomics: Past and Present

Steven Shorrock

> In this chapter:
> - A historical sketch of the beginnings of HF/E
> - Consideration of HF/E today and what needs to be done to improve HF/E integration in the near future

The Birth of a Discipline

During World War II, the United States lost hundreds of planes in accidents that were deemed 'pilot error'. Crash landings were a particular problem for the Boeing B-17 'Flying Fortress'. The planes were functioning as designed, and the pilots were highly trained, but made basic errors. In 1942, a young psychology graduate, Alphonse Chapanis, joined the Army Air Force (AAF) Aero Medical Lab as their first psychologist. Chapanis noticed that the flaps and landing gear had identical switches that were co-located and were operated in sequence. In the high-workload period of landing, pilots frequently retracted the gear instead of the flaps. This hardly ever occurred to pilots of other aircraft types. Chapanis fixed a small rubber wheel to the landing gear lever and a small wedge shape to the flap lever. This kind of 'pilot error' almost completely disappeared.

A few years later in 1947, experimental psychologists Paul Fitts and Richard Jones analysed accounts of 460 errors made in operating aircraft controls, through interviews and written reports. They noted that: 'It has been customary to assume that prevention of accidents due to material failure or poor maintenance is the responsibility of engineering personnel and that accidents due to errors of pilots or supervisory personnel are the responsibility of those in charge of selection, training, and operations.' Fitts and Jones took a different slant altogether. The basis for their study was the hypothesis that 'a great many accidents result directly from the manner in which equipment is designed and where it is placed in the cockpit'. What had been called 'pilot error' was actually a mismatch between characteristics of the designed world and characteristics of human beings, and between work-as-imagined and work-as-done (see Chapter 4).

Fitts and Jones considered a range of problems, including operating the wrong control, failing to adjust a control properly, forgetting to operate a control, moving a control in the wrong direction, unknowingly activating a control, and being unable to reach a control when needed. The flap–gear substitution error, and many other 'pilot errors', were actually problems of cockpit design. They concluded: 'Practically all pilots of present day AAF aircraft, regardless of experience or skill, report that they sometimes make errors in using cockpit controls. The frequency of these errors and therefore the incidence of aircraft accidents can be reduced substantially by designing and locating controls in accordance with human requirements'. They went on to specify design measures for controls and displays (concerning standardisation, simplification, sequencing, interlocks and other aspects of compatibility of controls with human characteristics and expectations).

These and other studies brought into focus the 'obvious fact' that human performance cannot be separated from the design of tasks, equipment and working environments. We can't just train and supervise human performance. We have to design for it. The studies and developments in this period are considered to be the birth of modern HF/E. Accidents associated directly with cockpit design are now extremely rare, and there has been a general decrease in commercial passenger fatalities even as air travel has increased. In fact, 2017 was the safest year on record, with no passenger deaths from flights in commercial passenger jets.

The Roots of HF/E

Prior to WWII, the roots of HF/E can be traced to various developments that were not related at the time, but provided an understanding of aspects of HF/E that are familiar today. This includes work carried out between the 15th and 19th centuries related to the study of human work, including physical exertion and fatigue, laws of time and motion, and the development of 'scientific management'. A more scientific approach to understanding human work emerged in the 19th and 20th centuries, occurring first in experimental psychology, especially from German psychologists. Subsequently, Frederick Taylor's 'time study' and Frank and Lillian Gilbreth's 'motion study' approaches emerged, based on observation, filming and analysis of human motion, using a special language and notation. These were combined into an approach that became known as 'time and motion study', and subsequently 'scientific management'. This was an approach to increasing productivity by scientific analysis of tasks, combined with selection, training, procedures, performance targets and measurement. Scientific management focused on efficiency of human work, including the study of skilled performance, in a range of contexts. However, Taylor and the Gilbreths did not see eye to eye. While this formed a first serious approach to the analysis of work, it was despised by trade unions, and in many ways left a bad legacy, for a number of reasons associated with how people were treated in terms of measurement, supervision, task design and – ultimately – automation. The focus of scientific management was on the productivity of human performance at the expense of the system as a whole, and human well-being. While time and motion study was very different to modern HF/E, observation and analysis remain key HF/E approaches.

In 1921 the National Institute of Industrial Psychology was formed in the UK – this made the results of experimental studies available to industry. Several other institutes followed over the subsequent decades. However, many would argue that research (in the USA and UK especially) concerning real work in real environments during and after WWII formed the beginnings of the discipline that came to be known as 'human factors' (USA) and 'ergonomics' (UK, and Europe, translated as appropriate). Research was primarily focused on selection and training, which places the emphasis on 'fitting the human to the task'. But during this period, the Oxford Climatic and Working Efficiency Research Unit was established. Cambridge University also constructed a unique cockpit research simulator known as the 'Cambridge Cockpit'. Studies in this simulator revealed the dependence of skilled behaviour on design, layout and interpretation of displays and controls. The need to fit the machine to the person, rather than vice versa, was realised. In parallel, Chapanis, Fitts and Jones uncovered the problems with aircraft displays and controls. Also in the 1940s, aviation psychology centres were established at Ohio State and Illinois Universities.

It was not the intention of early researchers to form a new discipline. Rather, 'the intention was much more modest, namely, to facilitate discussion, information exchange and collaboration between scientists working across a range of specialisms' (Waterson, 2016). These specialisms were anatomy, physiology, psychology, industrial medicine, industrial hygiene, design engineering, architecture and illumination engineering (Murrell, 1965).

The Growth of HF/E

Over time, HF/E became a distinct discipline. In 1949 the first book on HF/E, 'Applied Experimental Psychology: Human Factors in Engineering Design' was written by Chapanis, Garner and Morgan. The first society was the Ergonomics Research Society, which was formed in the UK in 1950 (now the Chartered Institute of Ergonomics and Human Factors), followed by the Human Factors Society of America in 1957 (now the Human Factors and Ergonomics Society). More research laboratories and units emerged in the military and in universities. Subsequently, more literature appeared (including the first journal – 'Ergonomics' – in 1957).

From this point on, HF/E developed both as a field of study and as a sphere of practice, and ultimately a profession. Between the 1960s and 1980s, HF/E grew rapidly, and became increasingly important in various sectors, especially the military and industry, and even space exploration. The HF/E societies grew in numbers. Short courses were developed, as well as the first undergraduate and postgraduate degrees. HF/E teams were set up in various industries, and consultancies emerged. Significantly, United Airlines set up a confidential incident reporting system. This was the basis for the FAA/NASA Aviation Safety Reporting System (ASRS). These initiatives helped to highlight the role of HF/E issues in aviation safety more generally.

In 1977, the worst aviation accident in history occurred: a runway collision at Tenerife, claiming 583 lives. Many factors were highlighted in the investigation

Chapter 2 – Human Factors and Ergonomics: Past and Present

that followed – none of which in isolation were sufficient to cause the accident. These included problems with pressure associated with duty-time regulations, communication (especially phraseology), procedures, decision making and team behaviour. In 1979, a major contained accident occurred at Three Mile Island nuclear power plant, Pennsylvania, USA. This revealed the potentially fatal consequences of poor control room design. During the 1980s, there were many more tragic disasters in high-hazard industries, including Chernobyl (Russia, nuclear power), Bhopal (India, chemical pesticide), Piper Alpha (Scotland, oil) and Challenger (USA, space). These all had consequences for the further development of HF/E.

HF/E in forensics and litigation became an important issue, and courts began to recognise HF/E issues in occupational and systems accidents. Control room design took increasing account of HF/E in the 1980s, and crew resource management (CRM) became established in airlines, and subsequently in other sectors. Human–computer interaction became a discipline and human–automation interaction became a new concern, and remains so today. More confidential HF/E reporting programmes were set up, including British Airways Safety Information System (BASIS) and Confidential Human Factors Incident Reporting Programme (CHIRP) in the UK.

In the 1990s, the safety case regime emerged in several countries, primarily as a result of the Piper Alpha oil disaster. Industry had to demonstrate that their operations were safe, and that risks were reduced 'as low as reasonably practicable' (ALARP) (further discussion on ALARP in Chapter 10). Occupational health and safety regulations were introduced in many countries. HF/E turned its attention increasingly towards air traffic management, rail, oil and gas, and chemical processing, paying particular attention to 'cognitive ergonomics', which is orientated to the psychological aspects of work both in how work affects the mind and how the mind affects work (Hollnagel 1997).

While HF/E was born partly from the study of accidents, it is important to emphasise that most research and application concerns everyday work, not accidents. Still, these and other accidents spurred research and practice in HF/E via funding and regulation, and recommendations from official inquiries that required the consideration of HF/E. The accidents have had implications for the entire scope of HF/E at three levels: micro (for example, display and control design), meso (for example, team interaction), and macro (for example, organisational processes and culture).

HF/E Development in Healthcare

In a book on human factors for paramedics, it may be notable that healthcare is missing from the brief historical sketch above. While HF/E is now increasingly a focus in healthcare, the uptake has been rather more significant in research than in practice.

As discussed in Chapter 1, the landmark report 'To Err is Human' was published in 1999. It was reported that up to 98,000 Americans were dying each year from 'medical errors'. Performance targets to reduce 'medical error' by 50% within five years were not achieved, despite media attention and US Congress calling for monitoring. The World Health Organization (WHO) has estimated that one in every 10 patients is harmed while receiving hospital care in high-income countries, with half or more of these considered preventable. Adverse events due to 'unsafe care' is likely to be one of the 10 leading causes of death and disability across the world, according to WHO, which estimates that harm to millions of patients, associated with unsafe medication practices, costs billions of US dollars.

So why has healthcare had a relatively weak influence on the development of HF/E as a discipline and profession? One reason may be how harm occurs in healthcare compared with other industries. In major hazard industries, such as oil and gas and aviation, people die in large numbers at one time when accidents occur, gaining much attention from media, public, politicians and regulators. In healthcare, people die one at a time over longer periods, even though the numbers are far greater for this sector than any other. This and other factors, such as problematic regulation, may be associated with a lack of uptake of HF/E in healthcare.

There are cases, however, where whole hospitals have been implicated in poor care. The inquiry into the UK Mid Staffordshire NHS Foundation Trust is a case in point. It has been estimated, based on a 2009 Healthcare Commission investigation, that hundreds of patients may have died as a result of poor care between 2005 and 2008 at Stafford Hospital. Performance targets and their influences on behaviour at all levels, from nurses to CEOs, were highlighted as negative influences in the Public Inquiry report by Robert Francis QC published on 6th February 2013. While this can be seen as a macro HF/E issue, the effect of the report on HF/E integration was small compared to major accidents such as the Tenerife runway accident or Piper Alpha oil platform fire, both of which were associated with hundreds of deaths.

HF/E as a discipline and profession has perhaps had the strongest impact in healthcare in research and in the design of medical devices. Researchers have focused on a range of issues, from the design of artefacts and environments to the assessment of safety culture. Practice has lagged behind, primarily due to the lack of full-time roles for qualified and experienced HF/E practitioners. One area of healthcare that has seen strong contributions from HF/E practice is the design of medical devices, though this has been done within private organisations, rather than in the National Health Service. Awareness among staff at all levels has, however, increased significantly with the help of the Clinical Human Factors Group (CHFG). The CHFG is a charity founded in 2007 by Martin Bromiley OBE, following the death of his wife Elaine Bromiley. Search online for 'just a routine operation' to watch filmed re-enactments of events that led to Elaine's death. The CHFG works with clinicians and experts to promote the use of HF/E to make healthcare safer for patients and staff, aiming to enhance understanding of HF/E in healthcare from board to ward and beyond. HF/E issues are now better understood, and many healthcare staff work in team training roles. However, specific roles for HF/E specialists to do the necessary design work remain rare, with fewer than 10 full-time (chartered, or similarly qualified and experienced) HF/E specialists in the NHS – an organisation of around 1.5 million staff (Shorrock, 2018).

Merging HF/E Today with Paramedic Context and Expertise

HF/E in practice today is a blend of applied science, engineering and craft. It cannot be argued to be any one of these exclusively. The approach tries to make system interaction and influence visible. It uses methods for data collection, analysis and synthesis to understand and map system interaction at every stage of the life cycle of a system or product. HF/E can therefore help in the design of interactions in the context of:

- artefacts (for example, equipment, signs, procedures, checklists)
- vehicles and designed environments (for example, ambulance layout, hospital design, lighting)
- task and job design (for example, pacing, timing, sequencing, variety, rostering, critical tasks)
- planned organisational activity (for example, supervision, training, regulation, handover, communication, scheduling, performance management)
- emergent aspects of organisations and groups (for example, culture, workload, trust, teamwork, relationships).

The contribution of HF/E as a discipline is primarily via theory and method, combined with the general orientation (see Chapter 1), especially the dual goals of optimising both system performance and human well-being, and the focus on system interactions (focus of understanding) and design (focus of intervention). However, this expertise is of little use in isolation. It needs to be combined with expertise in the work and the context of work, for example, paramedics, ambulance service provision and pre-hospital care. When combined, this 'emergent expertise' allows for good understanding and effective intervention. The HF/E approach may lead to the identification of a number of problems and opportunities, which can improve the pre-hospital system.

Types of 'Human Factors'

Over the last decade or so, the term 'human factors' has gained currency with an increasing range of people, professions, organisations and industries, especially in healthcare. It is a significant development, bringing what might seem like a niche discipline into the open, to a wider set of stakeholders. But as with any such development, there are inevitable differences in the meanings that people attach to the term, the mindsets that they bring or develop, and their communication with others. It is useful to know, then, what kind of 'human factors' we are talking about. At least four kinds seem to exist in our minds, each with somewhat different meanings and implications (see Shorrock, 2017).

1. **The Human Factor** – The first kind of human factors is the most colloquial: 'the human factor'. This seems to enter discussions about human and system performance in relation to unwanted events such as accidents. It is rarely defined explicitly, but tends to consider the human as a liability or unknown quantity. The term is rarely used by human factors specialists, and may be associated with the 'person-centred approach' to safety.

2. **Factors of Humans** – This kind of human factors focuses primarily on human characteristics, understood largely via reductionism (reducing people and systems down to 'components'). Factors of humans include, for example, cognitive functions and systems (such as memory, decision making), levels of performance (such as skill-based, rule-based and knowledge-based performance [Rasmussen, 1982]), error types (such as slips, lapses and mistakes [Reason, 1990]), physical functions and qualities, behaviours and skills, learning domains, and physical, cognitive and emotional states. These factors of humans may be seen as limitations and capabilities.

3. **Factors Affecting Humans** – This kind of human factors turns to the factors – external and internal to humans – that affect human performance: artefacts, organisational activity, environments, situations, job and work design, emergent aspects of organisations and groups, as well as aspects of human functions, qualities and states that affect performance (factors of humans). It is a broader focus which is common, but does not consider how humans affect systems.

4. **Socio-Technical System Interaction** – This kind of human factors aims to understand and design or influence purposive interaction between people and all other elements of socio-technical systems, concrete and abstract, at micro, meso and macro scales.

HF/E specialists should ultimately be concerned with the fourth kind of 'human factors' (which best reflects official definitions), but in light of the complexity of system performance and human well-being, the second and third kinds may be more evident in research and practice, and especially in communication with stakeholders, perhaps as deliberate simplifications (i.e. compromises and trade-offs).

Summary

The criticality of HF/E is not in dispute. For paramedic practice, HF/E offers an approach to understanding interactions between people and all other elements of a system, and to help design artefacts, vehicles and designed environments, tasks and jobs, and planned organisational activity. It also offers a way to understand emergent aspects of organisations and groups, prior to intervention.

So how to gain more traction on designing for human well-being and system performance? One way is to lobby for HF/E posts in organisations, including governmental organisations. Certain roles, typically involving a wide and deep level of content and method expertise, will always require highly qualified and experienced HF/E practitioners (for example, certified, registered, chartered).

Chapter 2 – Human Factors and Ergonomics: Past and Present

For instance, these specialists are now in higher demand, and having greater impact, in medical device design and pharmaceuticals. But this is only part of the solution. Healthcare has been reluctant to recruit HF/E specialists, perhaps without the regulatory requirements of high-hazard industries. So the other half of the solution is to spread HF/E to others, who might be familiar with certain aspects of HF/E theory and method, practising certain aspects of HF/E (for example, in the content or design of training), or advocating HF/E principles, but not HF/E specialists as such. This is where you come in. If the idea of designing for human use to optimise performance and human well-being appeals to you, then now is a good time to think about how you might learn more, and integrate HF/E in your practice.

References

Chapanis, A., Garner, W.R., Morgan, C.T. (1949). *Applied Experimental Psychology: Human Factors in Engineering Design*. New York: Wiley.

Fitts, P.M., Jones, R.E. (1947). *Analysis of Factors Contributing to 460 'Pilot Error' Experiences in Operating Aircraft Controls*. Dayton, OH: Aero Medical Laboratory, Air Material Command, Wright-Patterson Air Force Base.

Hollnagel, E. (1997). Cognitive ergonomics: it's all in the mind. *Ergonomics*. 40(10): 1170–1182.

Murrell, K.F.H. (1965). *Ergonomics: Man in his Working Environment*. London: Chapman and Hall.

Rasmussen, J. (1982). Human errors. A taxonomy for describing human malfunction in industrial installations. *Journal of Occupational Accidents*. 4(2–4): 311–333.

Reason, J. (1990). *Human Error*. Cambridge: Cambridge University Press.

Shorrock, S. (2017). Four kinds of human factors (series). Available from: https://humanisticsystems.com/2017/08/11/four-kinds-of-human-factors-1-the-human-factor/

Shorrock, S. (2018). The loneliest profession in healthcare. Available from: https://humanisticsystems.com/2018/05/11/the-loneliest-profession-in-healthcare/

Shorrock, S., Williams, C. (eds) (2016). *Human Factors and Ergonomics in Practice: Improving System Performance and Human Wellbeing in the Real World*. Boca Raton: CRC Press.

Waterson, P. (2016). 'Ergonomics and ergonomists: lessons for human factors and ergonomics practice from the past and present'. In: Shorrock S., Williams, C. (eds) (2016). *Human factors and ergonomics in practice: Improving System Performance and Human Wellbeing in the Real World*. Boca Raton: CRC Press.

Chapter 3
'Human Error'

Gary Rutherford

In this chapter:
- An introduction to some views on 'human error'
- Critique of the usefulness of the term and concept of 'human error'
- An example of a 'paramedic error' and how to look beyond it

Introduction

It is generally accepted that humans are fallible and will therefore make mistakes, and that these mistakes can occur in many ways in all aspects of life. The term 'human error' is commonly associated with, or attributed to, things going wrong or when there has been an unintended outcome. The 'To Err is Human' report mentioned in the preceding chapters suggests that 60–80% of adverse events in healthcare could involve 'human error'. In these circumstances the term is mainly used with good intent, to acknowledge that errors are normal, although it may also imply that a failure has been caused by the human (Woodward, 2019). This implication can also be seen in media report headlines following major accidents, where 'human error' can often be highlighted as the cause.

It is possible that when you started to read this book, you had anticipated more discussion on themes related specifically to human behaviour and performance, including 'human error', or its synonyms 'clinical error' or 'paramedic error'. However, hopefully by this stage of the book you have started to develop an appreciation that most incidents, accidents and things going wrong are systemic in origin and involve much more than just 'human error'.

'Human error' is mentioned in a few chapters of this book, and you may notice that it is presented within inverted commas. The purpose of this is to demonstrate scepticism of the term, which is a view held by most of the contributors of this text and provides a backdrop for the discussions in this chapter. In Chapter 2, the author mentions a couple of historical major incidents that have an element of 'human error',

Chapter 3 – 'Human Error'

and in another article, captures how the concept has been both a help and a hindrance to the development of HF/E:

> The popularisation of the term 'human error' has provided perhaps the biggest spur to the development of human factors in safety-related industries – with a downside. When something goes wrong, complexity is reduced to this simple, pernicious, term.
>
> (Shorrock, 2013)

This short chapter will explore the challenge of defining what 'human error' is, and discuss some viewpoints and theories. This will allow you to formulate your own thoughts on the value of the term 'human error' in paramedic practice, although it is likely to be clear that most of the contributors to this book find its value to be limited. It has been stated that 'errors cannot be eradicated' and that 'we can't fundamentally change the human condition, but we can change the conditions under which people work in order to make errors less likely' (Reason, 2008). Therefore, looking beyond 'human error' to understand the complex socio-technical system in everyday work is a theme throughout the book.

Defining 'Human Error'

'Human error' is a term that has created much debate for almost 50 years, with it becoming more commonly discussed after the nuclear reactor accident and subsequent radiation leak at Three Mile Island nuclear power plant in 1979 (Hollnagel, 2016), when workers did not recognise that a pressure relief valve was faulty. However, even after decades of significant research, there is still little agreement on what 'human error' means or how it can be defined (Shorrock, 2014a). One of the main issues is that 'human error' can have different meanings and be used in various ways. The term can be used to denote:

- the cause of something
- the event or action that occurred
- the outcome of the action.

A number of definitions attempt to incorporate one or more of these aspects. James Reason has been one of the leading cognitive psychologists to publish theories on 'human error', and he also recognises the lack of universally agreed definition (Reason, 2013). He suggests that most people acknowledge that some kind of 'deviation' is often involved, and proposed this definition:

> Error will be taken as a generic term to encompass all those occasions in which a planned sequence of mental or physical activities fails to achieve its intended outcome, and when these failures cannot be attributed to the intervention of some chance agency.
>
> (Reason, 1990)

Generally, 'human error' would seem to have evolved to imply a deviation of human performance from 'optimal' or 'correct' rules, procedures or actions. However, it could be suggested that for this type of view to hold true, there would need to be an understanding that an optimal or correct thing to do is clear or easily achievable, which is not always a strong feature of a complex system. Alternatively, strong views argue that the term is prejudicial, unspecific, and a socially constructed label that is proposed by others with hindsight after something has happened (Woods et al, 2010).

Types of Errors

There are a variety of subcategories and classifications of 'human error' that are suggested in order to try and explain or clarify meaning (Figure 3.1), and these can depend on the intention, the action, the outcome and the context of the error (Reason, 2008). 'Active errors' are proposed as those that are made by frontline workers, and are categorised and explained as:

- slips, trips and lapses — where a correct plan is devised, although actions do not go as planned, possibly due to absent-mindedness or clumsiness during implementation of the plan

- mistakes — when the plan is carried out exactly as was intended, however the plan was incorrect for the task required.

(Reason, 1997)

Incorporation of Rasmussen's (1983) three levels of performance — skill-based, rule-based and knowledge-based — offers further subcategorisation.

Dekker (2014) acknowledges the good intention of error categorisation tools and frameworks, highlighting how they aim to offer further explanation and understanding

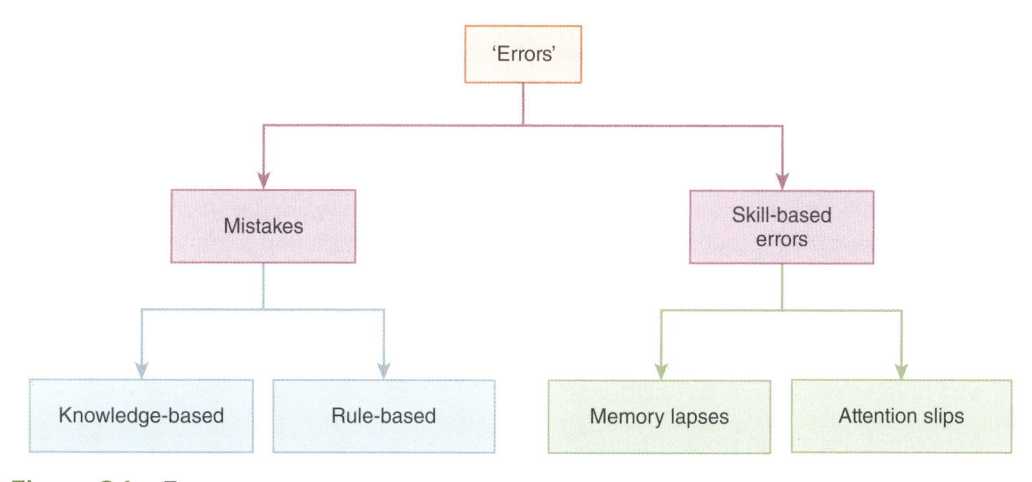

Figure 3.1 — Error types
Source: Based on Reason (1997) and Rasmussen (1983)

of what may have caused the error. After an incident, they can be used to 'probe the system for underlying reasons why it occurred' (Dekker, 2009). However, he goes on to suggest that this type of analysis oversimplifies the complexity of human behaviour within the system down to boxes, and may indicate that there is a quick fix. It is also suggested that labelling 'errors' merely identifies symptoms of the system function and malfunction, rather than any causes, and does not develop our understanding of how complex systems fail (Woods et al, 2010). Essentially, there are many types of error, however, the only way to differentiate them is with hindsight and knowledge of outcome. A paramedic may make the same decision or perform the same action frequently, although it would only be considered an 'error' where there is an undesired event or outcome.

Looking Beyond a 'Paramedic Error'

A pre-hospital example of the limitations and implications of identifying an incident as 'human error' could be when a 'drug error' is made by an ambulance clinician during the administration of medication to a patient. The commonly accepted pre-administration actions to be followed relate to the clinician checking that it is the right medication, including expiry date, right dose, right patient, to be given by the right route and for the right reasons (JRCALC, 2019). However, the lack of verification of these aspects is frequently cited as a 'root cause' of medication errors, leading to human failure as an explanation of this type of 'error'. This subsequently leads to the individual being given feedback to 'be more careful' in the future, and 'does not account for the sociotechnical nature of situated work' (Misasi and Keebler (2019). Many other system factors will likely have contributed to this type of 'error', such as similar medication packaging design and shared storage (see Figure 3.2 for potential examples of this), multiple tasks, poor guideline design and environmental conditions. These factors, along with inadequate lighting, distractions, stress, fatigue, steep authority gradients can all have an influence. Therefore, it becomes clearer how a conclusion of 'human error' is unlikely to minimise a future similar occurrence, and how it would be beneficial to look beyond this term. The design of equipment will be discussed further in Chapter 5.

Different Views of 'Human Error'

Dekker (2014) takes an approach to considering 'human error' that is helpful in diverting attention from the human to the system. He proposes that there are contrasting views of 'human error'; the 'old view' and a 'new view', with each significantly influencing the type of approach that is taken to carrying out reviews of when things go wrong and an 'error' has been made. An old view approach would believe that:

- complex system function is safe, it is unreliable people that are the problem
- 'human errors' cause accidents
- compliance with rules ensures safety
- when there is an unwanted outcome, people failed to do what they should have done.

Different Views of 'Human Error'

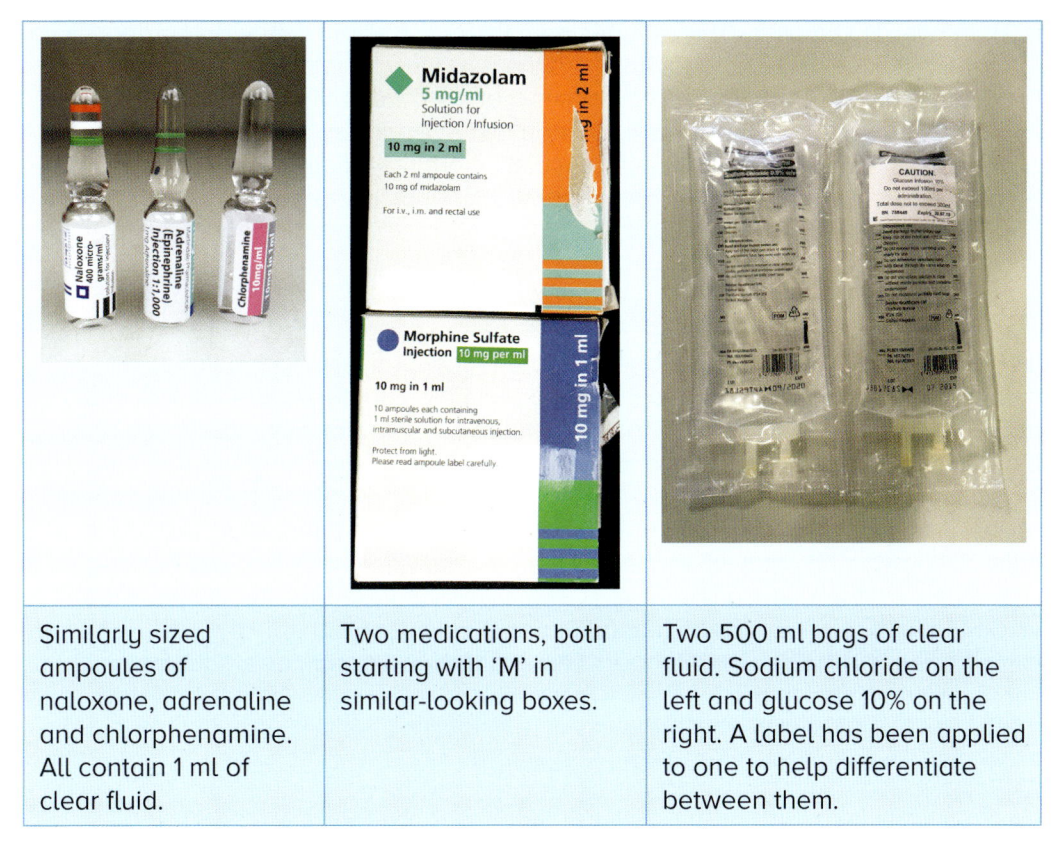

Similarly sized ampoules of naloxone, adrenaline and chlorphenamine. All contain 1 ml of clear fluid.	Two medications, both starting with 'M' in similar-looking boxes.	Two 500 ml bags of clear fluid. Sodium chloride on the left and glucose 10% on the right. A label has been applied to one to help differentiate between them.

Figure 3.2 – Similarities of medication packaging
Source: Images © Gary Rutherford

This approach can view the human as separate from the system, rather than being an integrated element of the work system, and consequently lead to 'human error' being a conclusion to an adverse event review. Subsequent person-centred recommendations can therefore be proposed, for example, re-training or advice for individuals to pay more attention or try harder to not make the same mistake again.

The alternative new view is to consider:

- that 'human error' is a symptom of issues with system functioning
- 'human error' as the starting point for a review, not a conclusion
- that 'human error' is systematically linked to tools, tasks and environments
- why people did what they did, and why it made sense at the time.

This new view supports the concept of adopting a systems approach to understanding when things have gone wrong in complex systems, to understand the conditions faced at the time, trying to avoid hindsight bias and knowledge of outcome.

Chapter 3 – 'Human Error'

Interestingly, Hollnagel (2016) critiques both the new and old views, and proposes an alternative 'no view'. He argues that even the new view maintains the term 'human error' as meaningful, and instead proposes that a 'no view' of 'human error' would demonstrate that it is not, and it should stop being used. He justifies this view by suggesting that all human activity is constantly variable, adjusting to conditions, and is never flawless. In this way 'errors' are part of normal, everyday work from which both wanted and unwanted outcomes emerge.

Summary

'Human error' is a term that has been debated for a long time, with a variety of theories and views that have been touched on in this chapter. Agreement on any definition that clearly explains what it is remains elusive. However, there may be benefit in professionals who have a duty of care to also have 'error wisdom' for circumstances known to provoke error (Reason, 2008). In relation to carrying out a review (see Chapter 10), 'human error' should never be the conclusion. Instead, it must be the starting point for the review.

While the term may have been helpful during the development of HF/E, its usefulness is now being increasingly challenged. The shortfalls of 'human error' can be summarised by stating that:

- it is usually a post hoc social judgement
- it requires a standard or specification that is incapable of being wrong
- it points to individuals in a complex system, where what we want to do is understand the system itself
- it stigmatises and scapegoats.

(Shorrock, 2014b)

As discussed in Chapters 1 and 2, HF/E is a design-driven discipline concerned with interacting elements within complex socio-technical work systems, of which the human is integral. Therefore, it can be a challenge to isolate 'human error' from the system. HF/E is not about eliminating 'human error', as this is impossible. One of the main purposes of HF/E is to enhance and strengthen system performance in order to avoid, reduce or mitigate 'human error' or its unwanted effects. Adopting a 'systems thinking' approach can help to facilitate this.

References

Dekker, S. (2009). Illusions of Explanation: a critical essay on error classification. *The International Journal of Aviation Psychology*. 13(2): 95–106.

Dekker, S. (2014). *The Field Guide to Understanding 'Human Error'*. 3rd Ed. Boca Raton: CRC Press.

Hollnagel, E. (2016). The NO view of 'human error' [online]. Available from: http://erikhollnagel.com/ideas/no-view-of-human-error.html

Joint Royal Colleges Ambulance Liaison Committee, Association of Ambulance Chief Executives (2019). *JRCALC Clinical Practice Guidelines 2019*. Bridgwater: Class Professional Publishing.

Misasi, P., Keebler, J.R. (2019). Medication safety in emergency medical services: approaching an evidence-based method of verification to reduce errors. *Therapeutic Advances in Drug Safety*. 10: 1–14.

Rasmussen, J. (1983). Skills, rules, and knowledge: signals, signs and symbols, and other distinctions in human performance models. *IEEE Transactions on Systems, Man, and Cybernetics*. SMC-13(3): 257–266.

Reason, J. (1990). *Human Error*. Cambridge: Cambridge University Press.

Reason, J. (1997). *Managing the Risks of Organizational Accidents*. Aldershot: Ashgate.

Reason, J. (2008). *The Human Contribution: Unsafe acts, accidents and heroic recoveries*. Farnham: Ashgate.

Reason, J. (2013). *A Life in Error: From little slips to big disasters*. Farnham: Ashgate.

Shorrock, S. (2013). 'Human Error': The handicap of human factors. *HindSight*. 18 [online]. Available from: https://www.skybrary.aero/index.php/Hindsight_18

Shorrock, S. (2014a). 'Human error': still undefined after all these years. *Humanistic Systems* [online]. Available from: https://humanisticsystems.com/2014/12/02/human-error-still-undefined-after-all-these-years/

Shorrock, S. (2014b). Life After Human Error. Keynote address from Velocity Europe 2014, Barcelona [online]. Available from: https://www.youtube.com/watch?v=STU3Or6ZU60

Woods, D.D. et al. (2010). *Behind Human Error*. 2nd Ed. Farnham: Ashgate.

Woodward, S. (2019). *Implementing Patient Safety: Addressing culture, conditions, and values to help people work safely*. Oxon: Routledge.

Chapter 4
Systems Thinking
Duncan McNab and Gary Rutherford

In this chapter:
- Definitions and types of systems
- Understanding the complex care system
- Tools to guide systems thinking approaches in pre-hospital care

Introduction

Systems thinking, or taking a systems approach, is key to achieving the dual aims of HF/E; improving system performance and optimising the well-being of both staff and patients. HF/E as a systems discipline 'examines, accounts for and enhances the design of a system, and people's interactions with it, rather than concentrating on an individual part of it' (Wilson, 2014). This supports Reason's (2000) assertion that adopting a systems approach to review adverse events may result in more learning and improvement than focusing on the actions of individuals.

As discussed in Chapters 1 and 2, HF/E and systems thinking are not just approaches to be adopted when something has gone wrong or there has been an adverse event. To understand a system with a view to improving its function, we need to analyse how everyday work happens, i.e. how the system operates under the different conditions likely to be faced. This everyday system operation is referred to as 'work-as-done' and understanding it is a key part of taking a systems thinking approach (EUROCONTROL, 2014). If the right kind of thinking is not adopted when considering system performance and human well-being, then understanding will be flawed and intervention ineffective (Shorrock, 2019).

Therefore, the focus of this chapter is to discuss what a systems approach is, and how it can be adopted and applied to understand and improve the way pre-hospital care systems work.

What is a System?

A system is 'an interconnected set of elements that is coherently organised in a way that achieves something' (Meadows, 2008). In Chapter 1, we considered

Chapter 4 – Systems Thinking

definitions of HF/E, and 'interactions among elements of a system' was highlighted as a key aspect. System elements can include people, tasks, equipment and work environments that continuously interact with each other in various ways to achieve a shared purpose.

The benefits of systems of care are increasingly recognised in pre-hospital care, with improved clinical outcomes for patients being demonstrated when elements of work systems are designed to interact effectively, and when related systems interact with each other. Examples can be seen in the management of out-of-hospital cardiac arrest (Scottish Government, 2019) and the establishment of major trauma systems (Moran et al, 2018).

Types of Systems

There are many types of systems across society, although they can generally be categorised as:

- simple
- complicated
- complex.

(Glouberman and Zimmerman, 2002)

Simple Systems

A simple system is usually one that is predictable and easy to understand. An example of one is a recipe for making a cake. The recipe will have some specific elements relating to technique and terminology, however, even without any particular expertise, following the steps will produce results with a reasonable chance of success (Glouberman and Zimmerman, 2002). In these types of systems it is generally easy to break down each step and analyse what would happen if components were omitted, substituted or re-ordered.

Complicated Systems

In complicated systems there are lots of interacting components, and they can contain subsets of simple systems (Glouberman and Zimmerman, 2002). Despite this, it is normally possible to break the system down into its individual components, and determine how each works and the effect of the performance of that component on the overall system. Technical and mechanical equipment are often considered as examples of complicated systems, with engines and gearboxes commonly used to illustrate this (Figure 4.1). Although the intricate working is likely to be too complicated for most of us to understand, engineers and mechanics can dismantle this type of system to inspect and analyse the operation and serviceability of each component. Simple and complicated systems are both usually predictable and understood by taking them apart. When things go wrong, the faulty element can usually be identified and replaced, allowing the system to return to normal function.

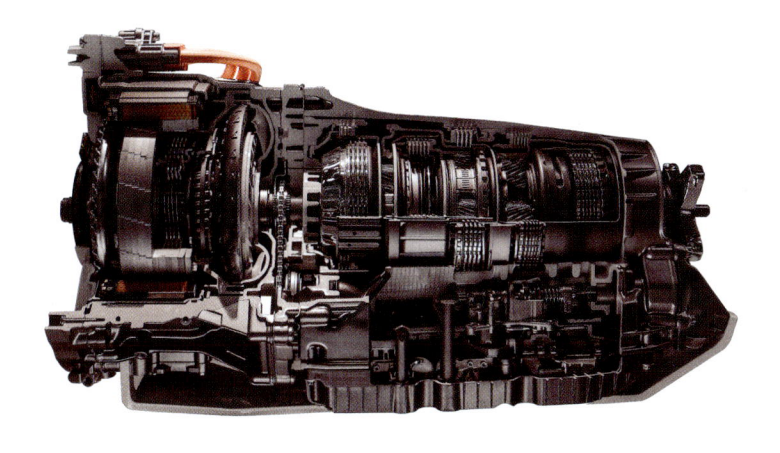

Figure 4.1 – Car gearbox
Source: Shutterstock by patruflo

Complex Systems

The terms 'complicated' and 'complex' can often be used interchangeably, however, there are significant differences when applied to the understanding of systems. Complex systems are not constructed in the same way as complicated ones. They tend to grow or evolve over a significant period of time rather than being constructed to a plan. They can be very dynamic, where the interacting elements simultaneously affect and are shaped by the system. In such systems, conditions can change rapidly and often in an unpredictable way, with unexpected events occurring. Therefore, they can be very difficult to break down for analysis and prediction of performance.

Organisations, such as healthcare, are examples of complex systems (Carayon, 2006). Emergency medical services can therefore also be considered complex systems, although each one is unique (Resuscitation Academy, 2018). These types of systems consist of technical elements such as tools, equipment, information and communication technology, policies and processes, although the added elements of services users, management teams and frontline workers make it a complex socio-technical system (Johns, 2019).

Understanding Complex Care Systems

Complex care systems possess a number of characteristics that can be recognised in ambulance services:

- A large number of dynamically interacting elements are present.
- Any element in the system is affected by and affects other elements or systems.

Chapter 4 – Systems Thinking

- Small changes can lead to large effects, due to the non-linear interactions.
- Challenges are encountered in defining system boundaries.
- Energy is required to maintain the system organisation.
- Historical events influence and shape present system function.

(The Health Foundation, 2010)

There are numerous systems that interact with each other in pre-hospital care: control centres, ambulance stations, ambulance vehicles, treatment and management plans, each with their own subsystems. These are all also influenced by performance or changes in other parts of healthcare systems such as GPs, out-of-hours services, emergency departments, hospital wards and other emergency and social care services. Small changes to system element interactions can cause large effects in other parts of the system. For example, phrasing one key question in a different way during the telephone triage processes in ambulance control centres may cause a significant impact on the triage category and subsequent ambulance response.

This complexity means that it can be difficult to understand how safety is created and maintained within a complex system. To gain a better understanding of complex systems, it is essential to consider the purpose of the overall system and the effect on that purpose of the interactions between components. A key aspect is to accept that things going well or going wrong can emerge from the same dynamic work system interactions and processes that are occurring all the time, i.e. everyday work. These 'interactions' and 'processes' may be considered rather nebulous terms that don't offer clear direction on what to look for and how to understand complex system performance and behaviour. Therefore, to take a systems approach within complex care systems, methods are needed that look beyond individual components of care, to explore and understand how everyday work occurs (McNab et al, 2020).

Work-as-Done vs Work-as-Imagined

Due to the continually changing challenges faced in complex systems, it is often not possible to fully specify, or describe, 'work'. Shorrock (2017) discusses how understanding and improving human work within a system can be difficult for those who design and do the work. He highlights a long-standing simple concept that 'how people think that work is done and how work is actually done are two different things' as a useful way of considering complex human work. These views of the work system are known as work-as-imagined and work-as-done, and are described further in Table 4.1.

Work-as-imagined is a view that is often held by those who do not do the work. This is commonly described as how managers believe frontline work is done, although can also relate to how frontline staff think managers do their work. In contrast, work-as-done is the actual everyday work by those who do the work. Understanding work-as-done, and the gaps between it and work-as-imagined, are essential to systems thinking and design (EUROCONTROL, 2014).

Understanding Complex Care Systems

Table 4.1 – Descriptions of work-as-imagined and work-as-done

Type of Work	Description
Work-as-imagined	This is the work that we imagine that others do and the work that we do, both now and in the future. Often our imagination of how others do their work is incorrect or inaccurate. Similarly, it is likely that how we imagine we would do something is different from how we actually do it.
Work-as-done	This is the actual work activities that occur, and usually in a different way to imagined. It can often be achieved by the worker making adjustments, trade-offs and workarounds to get the job done to meet demand.

Workarounds and Trade-Offs

Despite the complexity, healthcare goes right most of the time and this is often due to the people who work in the system. Workers on the frontline often adapt how they perform a task in order to get the work done. These adaptations are referred to as workarounds and trade-offs, and are frequently performed in good faith during everyday work, although they can be viewed negatively by others with hindsight when things go wrong.

A workaround is when a standard way of working is changed to cope with the conditions faced. Workaround behaviours or actions can be applied to circumvent a 'problem' in rule, process or workflow design (Debono et al, 2013). Trade-offs are situational decisions where one aspect is sacrificed in order to achieve gains in another. These trade-off decisions and behaviours can often be made between efficiency and thoroughness or between short- and long-term goals (Hollnagel, 2009). Efficiency usually involves completing a task using as little resource as possible, and in contrast thoroughness involves taking great care, attention to detail and sufficient time to complete a task successfully.

Examples of workarounds by ambulance clinicians:

- To assist with the safe administration of injectable medication, the application of sticky identification labels to syringes containing drawn up drugs is recommended (Crossman, 2009). However, if these labels have not been introduced to the system or are unavailable, clinicians may 'work around' this by applying tape to the syringes, using different sized syringes for different drugs or keeping multiple syringes apart.

- Some ambulance services provide a telemetry system for decision making support related to electrocardiograph (ECG) interpretation. If technical difficulties are encountered related to transmission of the ECG directly from the machine, ambulance clinicians may work around this by utilising other technical solutions, for example use of WhatsApp, multimedia or text message to send the ECG to a device in the receiving centre, despite the risk that this may breach information governance policies.

Chapter 4 – Systems Thinking

- Restocking ambulance consumables from hospital departments and wards may also be a workaround of barriers to recommended or desired restocking processes. For example, if an ambulance crew administer their only dose of heparin to a patient, they may be able to obtain a replacement dose from the receiving unit so that they are not without one until they return to station (or they know that none are available on station). However, this may risk the incorrect strength of heparin being inadvertently introduced to the system.

Ambulance clinicians are also faced with situations that require efficiency–thoroughness trade-offs. For example, if there is a requirement to move a bariatric patient during a clinically urgent situation, additional colleagues would ideally be available to assist with moving and handling. However, a trade-off decision may be made by the two-person crew to move the patient themselves, which increases the personal injury risk but reduces the clinical risk to the patient that may be associated with waiting for additional help. Efficiency–thoroughness trade-offs may also occur during the completion of patient care record documentation, where the requirement to record and document as much detail as possible (thoroughness) may be desired, although must be balanced with time pressure to be ready for the next call (efficiency).

Ambulance control centres are also systems where call handling and dispatch staff are often required to employ workarounds and efficiency–thoroughness trade-offs. Workarounds may be required to manually prioritise between multiple calls in response to the algorithmic triage process indicating that they are the same category. Trade-offs may also be required when managing the demands on resources, for example, the number of emergency calls waiting to be answered (efficiency) versus the time that can be spent remaining on the call offering further support and guidance to the caller (thoroughness).

It is possible that these examples may be considered by some to be instances of poor practice, however, in reality they are normal 'work-as-done' situations that usually result in good outcomes and increased efficiency. Understanding these situations and using this understanding to address system problems and subsequently close the gaps between 'work-as-done' and 'work-as-imagined' will lead to strengthening of the system.

'Human Error' vs 'Systems Thinking'

As described in Chapter 3, the use of the term 'human error' is contentious. When there is an unwanted outcome (such as a patient suffering harm), it can be a natural response to work backwards from that event and look for, and find, something that people did 'wrong' – for example, not following protocols. But unless we understand work-as-done, what was happening at the time (the system conditions) and why people made the decisions they did, they will be required to use the same workarounds and make the same trade-offs when similar circumstances re-occur. What we rarely do is work backwards from successful events. If we do that, again, we often find things that people have done 'wrong', but these have led to good outcomes. In addition, sometimes people do exactly as they are supposed to do and still there is an unwanted outcome. A 'systems approach' helps us to move beyond blaming 'human error' to understand why decisions made sense at the time and then to design system improvements to support the work of staff in challenging or changing conditions.

Frameworks to Guide Systems Thinking

Tools are available that can help us to understand the workings of a complex system and guide us to adopt a systems approach during analysis. This can be retrospective, when things have gone wrong (or gone well), and also when prospectively considering system function. Two models based on HF/E principles will be considered; the Systems Engineering Initiative for Patient Safety (SEIPS) and the Systems Thinking for Everyday Work (STEW) models that were introduced in Chapter 1.

SEIPS

The SEIPS model (Figure 4.2) defines and illustrates what can be considered when thinking about the interacting elements, outcomes and design of a healthcare system. It utilises a structure-process-outcome quality improvement framework to present an HF/E approach to healthcare systems thinking. The left-hand side of the model, the 'work system', presents the interactions between five main proposed elements of a system, i.e. the person(s), the tasks involved, the variety of tools and technologies that may be used, and the environment and organisational conditions in which they occur. Carayon (2006) and Holden et al (2013) describe each element:

- **Person** – including both healthcare professionals and patients. The person element is deliberately placed in the centre of the work system to highlight how people are central in healthcare and to the design of the work system. Factors to consider related to the person are the skills, experience and requirements of the healthcare professional, and the preferences, goals and needs of the patient.
- **Tasks** – that the healthcare professional carries out, focusing on the characteristics of the task, for example, difficulty, complexity and variety.
- **Tools and technologies** – for example, medical devices, equipment, and information and communication technologies.
- **Environment** – related to the physical aspects such as lighting, temperature, noise and physical layout.
- **Organisation** – refers to elements such as policies and procedures, work schedules, training programmes, culture and resource availability.

These work system elements can interact with each other, often with multiple simultaneous interactions occurring. Understanding this interaction between elements is a strong theme when taking an HF/E approach to considering system function. The interactions within the work system influence how care is provided and this is presented in the 'process' section of care delivery. The processes are

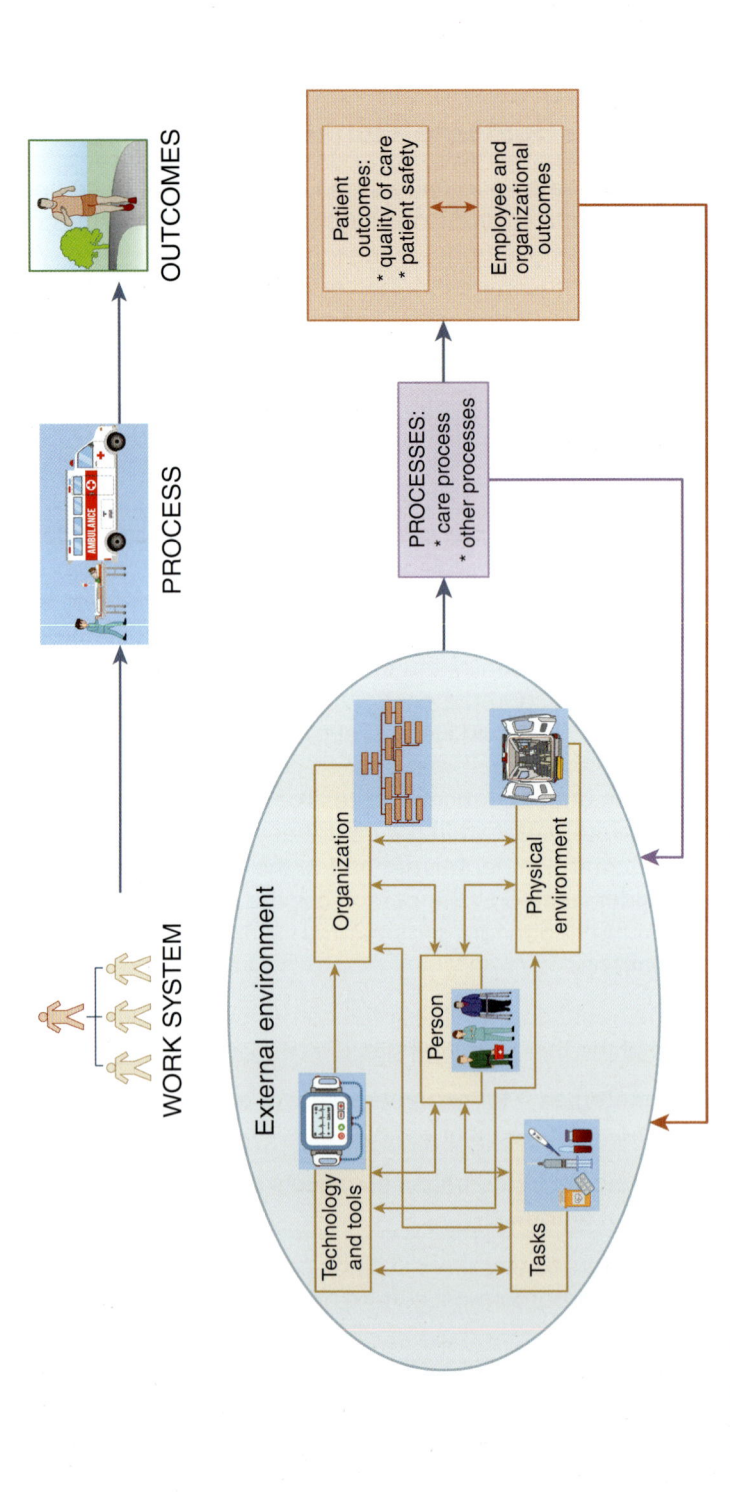

Figure 4.2 – Systems Engineering Initiative for Patient Safety

Source: Reproduced from Work system design for patient safety: the SEIPS model, Carayon et al, 15(Suppl 1), i51, 2006 with permission from BMJ Publishing Group Ltd

the actual treatment plans and support mechanisms that have been shaped by the work system, for example, pre-hospital treatment or referral to another part of the healthcare system. The patient can also be involved in these care processes. The 'outcomes' part illustrates the potential and actual desirable and undesirable outcomes that can result for patients, staff and healthcare organisations, i.e. patient safety, staff outcomes (well-being, job satisfaction) and system performance (organisational outcomes). Importantly, this model also proposes that the learning from these processes and outcomes should be fed back and used to adapt, strengthen and re-design the work system.

To consider this model further, we can apply it to a particular system within pre-hospital care and contrast it with a simple system view.

SEIPS Applied to Out-of-Hospital Falls Pathways

Calls for people over 65 years of age who have fallen are one of the most common requests to ambulance services, comprising 10–25% of ambulance attendances to this age group (JRCALC, 2019). This has led to increased focus on appropriately managing these patients, particularly those who could benefit from intervention and support from community health and social care teams, in order to minimise future falls. This is usually done by implementation of 'falls referral pathways' which can have variable success (Mikolaizak et al, 2016; Snooks et al, 2017).

Figure 4.3 demonstrates a simple, linear system view of the processes and interacting elements related to an ambulance call to a person who has fallen and the subsequent triage decisions. Application of the SEIPS model to the same work system (Figure 4.4) allows more dynamic illustration and deeper consideration of the interacting and influencing elements of this complex work system.

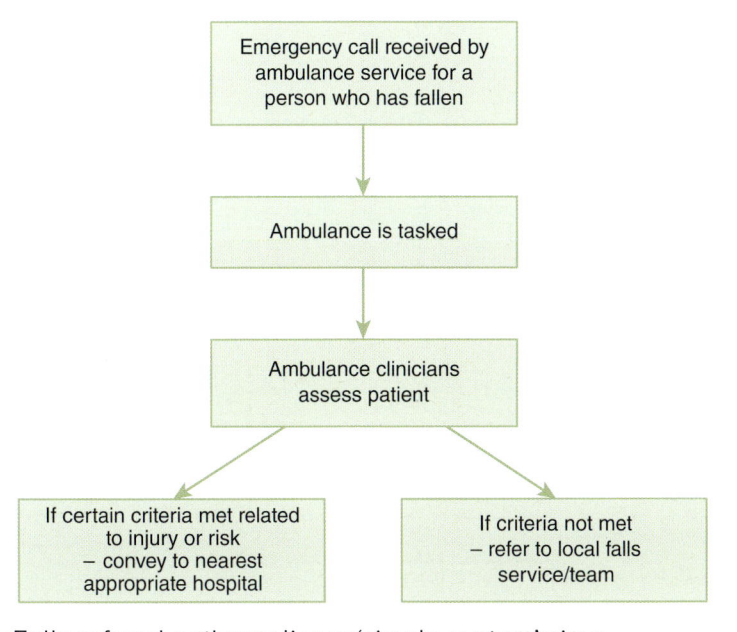

Figure 4.3 – Falls referral pathway linear 'simple system' view

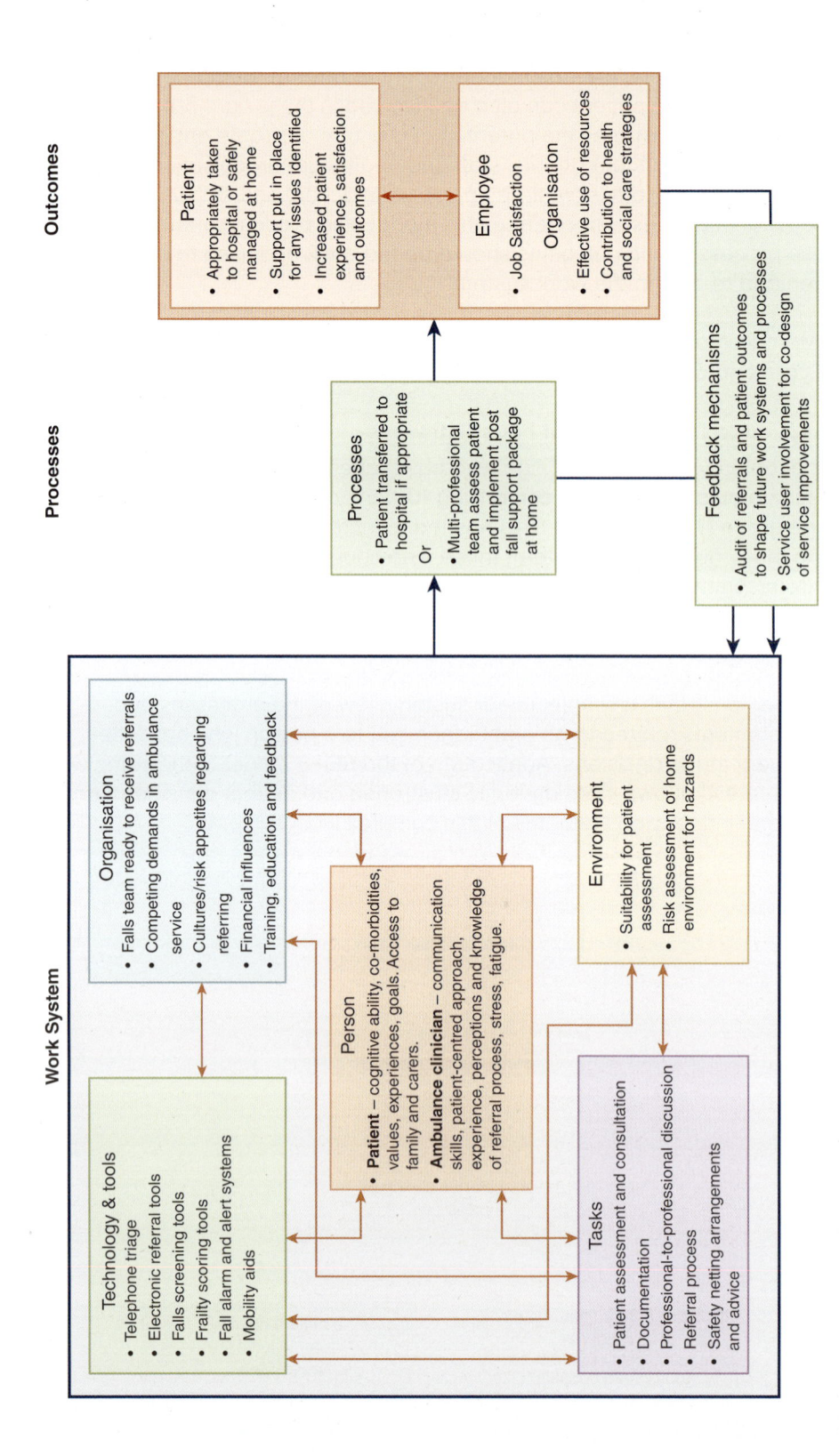

Figure 4.4 – SEIPS model applied to systems for 'falls'

A 'non-systems approach' to improving compliance with falls referral protocols may be to put posters or bulletins on noticeboards in ambulance stations to advise clinicians of the process that should be followed, and criticise the individuals when they don't do it. Conversely, adopting a systems approach and applying a tool to consider the multiple interacting components that influence performance may assist in understanding how to implement change to produce desired outcomes. The understanding of these interactions and outcomes should make it easier to do the 'right thing'.

Systems Thinking for Everyday Work (STEW)

The previously described SEIPS model predominantly helps to define and describe the interacting elements within the work system, which can be helpful in ensuring a systems approach rather than a person-focused one. To explore further how work actually happens in these systems, other models can be helpful. A framework for understanding performance in complex systems was developed by EUROCONTROL (a European air traffic management organisation) and presented in their white paper 'Systems Thinking for Safety: Ten Principles' (2014). These principles were adapted for use in healthcare by a group of frontline healthcare professionals and national safety leaders in Scotland to produce the Systems Thinking for Everyday Work (STEW) model (Figure 4.5). The STEW model can be utilised to structure a team-based discussion or to guide individuals who are commissioned to carry out a review. It consists of a foundation concept and five interlinked principles, which can help to:

- understand the current system
- analyse incidents (with both wanted and unwanted outcomes)
- identify improvement priorities
- develop 'change ideas' and their implementation into current work systems
- monitor, evaluate and spread change.

(McNab et al, 2020)

The foundation concept prompts us to consider the system as a whole rather than focusing on individual components. For practical purposes, to analyse a system it is usually beneficial to agree the boundary for the review. This can be challenging as the boundary is not normally real, and that work is influenced by factors outside this boundary, i.e. other systems or system elements. Wilson (2014) discusses the challenges of identifying where one system ends and another begins, for the purposes of analysis. Therefore, boundaries should just be as sensible and clear as possible to allow a meaningful and helpful analysis to be carried out. The model encourages engagement with those doing the work, to gain multiple perspectives to help understand how system conditions and performance are perceived by those within it. Where appropriate, it may be beneficial to seek and include the views of the patient or service user. Work conditions include consideration of demand, capacity, resources and constraints. Analysing interactions and workflow within the system involves considering interactions between people, tasks, equipment and

Chapter 4 – Systems Thinking

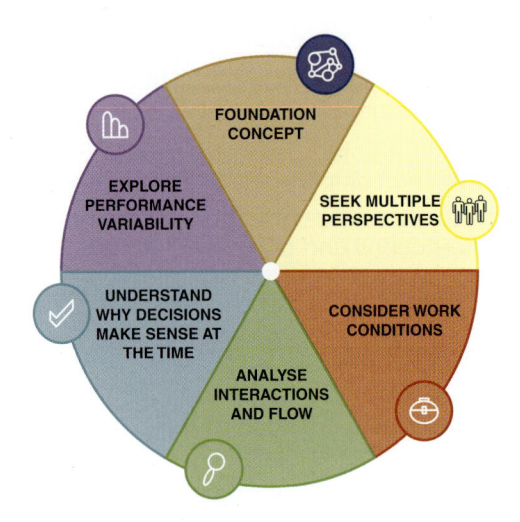

Figure 4.5 – Systems Thinking for Everyday Work
Source: NHS Education for Scotland (2018). Reproduced with permission

the environment, as well as policies that may cause bottlenecks and blockages. This can lead to an understanding of why people make the decisions they do, how people adapt to different conditions to continue to achieve success, and can help to avoid hindsight bias and blaming 'human error'. In this way we can get closer to understanding work-as-done, and the associated workarounds and trade-offs that are needed to adapt to changing work conditions.

The optimal way to apply STEW in practice would be in a facilitated group or team discussion, to promote deeper understanding of the system using each of the principles, further illustrated in Figure 4.6.

STEW Applied to a Pre-Hospital Case

STEW can be utilised to consider a range of paramedic practice or ambulance service situations and work systems. Possible systems to consider could be implementation of new care pathways, reviews of existing ones, handover processes, delays at hospital, call handling and resource dispatch processes, professional-to-professional support, non-conveyance decisions, triage decisions, and multi-agency incident responses. We will consider STEW in the analysis of a case in keeping with the falls theme in this chapter. In Box 4.1 is the initial '1st story' related to a patient who sustained an injury from a fall, a few hours after a paramedic had attended to them and agreed they could remain at home. This could be an example of a case where it might be easy to slip into conducting a person-focused review rather than a system-focused one. A 1st story is the quickly emerging account of an incident, that often focusses on individuals involved. The 2nd story usually takes longer to compile, presents wider system issues and normally requires to be actively sought (see Chapter 10 for more discussion on 1st and 2nd stories). Table 4.2 illustrates how the principles of STEW could be applied to explore the '2nd story' for this case, with example questions and elements for group consideration and discussion.

1. Foundation Concept

Consider the overall system rather than focusing on isolated parts, events or outcomes.

- Agree boundaries.
- Agree purpose of system and parameters for success.

2. Seek Multiple Perspectives

Appreciate that people at all levels are local experts in the work that they do.

- Recognise that different people, in different roles will have different perspectives.
- Explore the experiences and views of all people who work in the system to better understand the work system and change implementation issues.

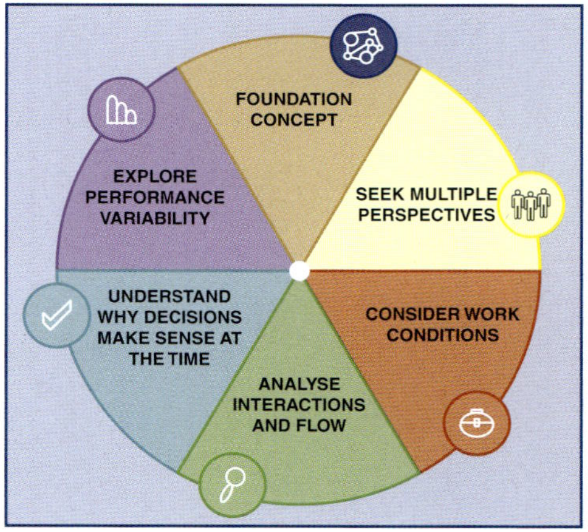

3. Consider Work Conditions

Appreciate that the interacting combination of demand, capacity, resource availability and constraints influences the way that people undertake work at any given time.

- Explore and understand how demand varies over time and if this variation is matched by changes in capacity.
- Where feasible ensure essential resources are available.
- Identify leading indicators of impending trouble by anticipating changes in conditions.
- Examine how work conditions affect staff well-being (e.g. health, safety, motivation, job satisfaction) and performance (care quality, safety, productivity, effectiveness).

4. Analyse Interactions and Work Flow

Appreciate that interactions between people, tasks, equipment, environments and external influences are complex and dynamic.

- When making changes consider the impact on overall system functioning.
- Explore how system interactions affect patient or information flow.

5. Understand Why Decisions Make Sense at the Time

When looking back on individual, team or organisational decision-making, appreciate that people do what makes sense to them based on the system conditions experienced at the time.

- Explore how conditions, interactions and personal and team goals at the time influenced decisions.
- Be wary of hindsight bias.
- Avoid blaming 'human error' and promote a 'just culture' - understand what happened, support those involved and improve work systems to reduce the risk of recurrence.

6. Explore Performance Variability

People constantly have to vary how they do work to achieve successful outcomes due to changing system conditions.

- Acknowledge that work conditions change rapidly, so adjustments are needed for success.
- Consider how workarounds and trade-offs contribute to successful and unsuccessful outcomes.
- Explore the difference between work-as-imagined and work-as-done.
- Appreciate that desired and undesired outcomes often emerge from the same source – everyday work.

Figure 4.6 – STEW principles for use during group discussions

Source: NHS Education for Scotland (2018). Reproduced with permission

Chapter 4 – Systems Thinking

> **Box 4.1 – Fall Patient Not Referred '1st Story'**
>
> A 72-year-old male, Harry, fell at home one afternoon and was unable to get up. He was able to alert a neighbour and a single response paramedic subsequently attended. The paramedic assessed Harry and no injury was identified. Harry recalls falling, stated that he was not sure what happened but was certain that he did not feel unwell prior to the fall. The paramedic assisted Harry to his feet, who was able to weight bear and mobilise to a different room in the house although he remained unsteady. Harry described a past medical history of angina, had a similar fall about 6 weeks ago, and stays on his own after his wife died 2 years ago. He does not have any personal care package, but receives almost daily visits from family members.
>
> A local falls pathway was recently established in Harry's area, although the paramedic did not make a referral during this care episode. Harry was reluctant to be referred, instead stating a preference to discuss things further with his daughter who was expected to visit him later that day. The paramedic phoned the daughter but got no response; a neighbour arrived and said he could sit with Harry for an hour and that the daughter always visited that night of the week and was probably on her way.
>
> Harry had another fall in the evening of the same day. His daughter had not been able to drop in to see him as expected, so he lay on the floor all night until found by another family member the next morning. An ambulance attended and he was suspected to have sustained a fractured neck of femur.

Table 4.2 – Questions to guide a systems approach using STEW to explore the 2nd story

Principles and Questions	Specific Elements to Consider
Foundation Concept • What is the overall purpose of the system you are considering? • Where would you set the boundaries for reviewing the system(s) that you are thinking of? You need to find a balance with considering the overall care system and the practicality of reviewing what you can influence. • What does optimal system performance or success look like?	To minimise unnecessary conveyance and admission to hospital? To minimise the risk of future falls? To decrease the number of falls calls to the ambulance service? Does the boundary include ambulance control centres, or other health and social care services?

(continued)

Table 4.2 – Questions to guide a systems approach using STEW to explore the 2nd story *(continued)*

Principles and Questions	Specific Elements to Consider
Seek multiple perspectives • Who needs to be involved in the review, from all levels, to ensure that all elements of the work system are represented and understood?	Frontline ambulance clinicians, community health and social care colleagues, secondary care colleagues, patient/representatives, QI (Quality Improvement) or HF/E specialist support, ICT advisors?
Consider work conditions • What are/were the work conditions that need to be considered? • How does demand on the system vary and is there capacity to cope with additional demand? • What are the main constraints to system success in relation to the conditions? • How do these factors affect staff well-being and performance?	Do ambulance clinicians have access to up-to-date Emergency Care Summaries related to patients? Do they have access to telephone numbers for local falls support services? Do falls support services have capacity to attend or assist? What had been the demands on this paramedic during this shift? Tired, hungry, stressed – affecting decision making. Knowledge, access and usability of guidelines regarding referral process to be followed in this area. Was the paramedic working in their normal geographical area?
Analyse interactions and workflow • What are the key interactions? • Do people interact with each other and is this optimal? • Do people interact with equipment, technology, SOPs (standard operating procedures), guidelines, and have these things been designed for people to use with ease? • Are there any external regulations that enhance or hinder system performance? • If you make changes to a part of the system, what other parts do you anticipate being affected?	Were shared decision-making techniques adopted with patient and family? Ease of access to professional-to-professional decision-making support. Increased job cycle time if referral processes are inefficient.

(continued)

Chapter 4 – Systems Thinking

Table 4.2 – Questions to guide a systems approach using STEW to explore the 2nd story (*continued*)

Principles and Questions	Specific Elements to Consider
Understand why decisions make sense at the time • Put yourself in the position of the person who made the decision at that time with the information that they had, and not knowing the outcome that is known at the time of the review. Are you avoiding hindsight bias? • Does this help highlight system vulnerability? • Are you avoiding saying 'human error' was the cause? • Are you promoting a just culture, i.e. not punishing for actions in line with experience and training?	Harry's desires and wishes may have been met. It seemed a safe decision at the time to leave Harry as his daughter would soon be there. Decision only now seems flawed with knowledge that Harry later fell again. If the daughter had arrived and Harry had not fallen this would have been described as good care as it kept Harry out of hospital. Blaming this paramedic will not enhance (and will likely inhibit) future use of referral pathways.
Explore performance variability • Have any trade-offs or workarounds been applied to achieve goals? • Can the system be adapted to minimise high-risk trade-off and workaround requirements of people? • Is there a gap between work-as-imagined (WAI) and work-as-done (WAD)? • How can any gap be addressed?	This paramedic may have worked around Harry's reluctance for referral by agreeing to his request to discuss with daughter. They also left the neighbour with Harry. If a referral pathway exists, WAI by management is that the referral would always be made. WAD is therefore different. Explore to understand why WAD differs from WAI.

Utilisation of frameworks for structuring a systems thinking approach is beneficial, however, it is emphasised that it is the 'insights, understandings and perspectives that emerge along the way from conversation' that are most important (Shorrock, 2019). The STEW model encourages an exploration of these factors and is a helpful tool to guide a systems approach to understanding how normal, everyday work takes place within a system.

Summary

Taking a systems approach is a fundamental principle of HF/E. It promotes a deeper exploration of system functioning which is essential for learning from challenging situations and everyday work, including when things go well. Understanding the work system interactions of everyday 'work-as-done' is key. It can be difficult to know where to start when analysing complex system function. The included frameworks help define what a 'systems approach' actually entails and how it can be applied within the pre-hospital context to facilitate conversations and identify improvement opportunities.

The SEIPS model describes the interactions between components and processes within the system, while the STEW model explores *how* these interactions influence everyday work within the system, thereby complementing use of the SEIPS model. Although standardising and simplifying processes is important within HF/E, in a resource-limited environment, it will never be possible to fix all system problems or consider all conditions that will be faced. Therefore, the contribution of humans to creating safety needs to be explored, understood and enhanced. Understanding how safety is created and maintained must involve more than examining when it fails. Both models presented can be used prospectively to explore system functioning with a view to improvement before an unwanted event occurs.

A conscious effort to adopt systems thinking will allow a deeper and more comprehensive approach to problem-solving, managing change and planning ahead. It will also minimise the identification of 'human error' as the cause of unintended outcomes, and instead will encourage the design of improvement interventions to the benefit of the patient, ambulance clinician and pre-hospital organisation. Not only will this improve outcomes but will support staff by avoiding unwarranted blame.

In the next chapters of this book, the key interacting elements and design of the pre-hospital work system will be discussed in further detail, considering equipment and process design, the patient, the ambulance clinician (as an individual and in teams), learning from events and safety culture.

References

Carayon, P. (2006). Human factors of complex sociotechnical systems. *Applied Ergonomics*. 37(4): 525–535.

Carayon, P. et al. (2006). Work system design for patient safety: the SEIPS model. *Quality & Safety in Health Care*. 15(Suppl 1): i50–i58.

Crossman, M. (2009). Technical and environmental impact on medication error in paramedic practice: a review of causes, consequences and strategies for prevention. *Journal of Emergency Primary Health Care*. 7(3): 1–10.

Debono, D.S. et al. (2013). Nurses' workarounds in acute healthcare settings: a scoping review. *BMC Health Services Research*. 13: 175.

EUROCONTROL (2014). Systems Thinking for Safety: Ten Principles (a white paper) [online]. Available from: https://www.skybrary.aero/bookshelf/books/2882.pdf

Glouberman, S., Zimmerman, B. (2002). Complicated and complex systems: what would successful reform of Medicare look like? In: *Romanow Papers: Changing Health Care in Canada* (Vol. 2). Forest, P.-G., Marchildon, G.P., McIntosh, T. (eds). Toronto: University of Toronto Press.

Holden, R.J. et al. (2013). SEIPS 2.0: a human factors framework for studying and improving the work of healthcare professionals and patients. *Ergonomics*. 56(11): 1669–1686.

Chapter 4 – Systems Thinking

Hollnagel, E. (2009). *The ETTO Principle: Efficiency-thoroughness Trade-off: Why things that go right sometimes go wrong*. Farnham: Ashgate.

Johns, A. (2019). Complicated and complex systems in safety management [online]. Available from: https://www.linkedin.com/pulse/complicated-complex-systems-safety-management-adam-johns

Joint Royal Colleges Ambulance Liaison Committee, Association of Ambulance Chief Executives (2019). *JRCALC Clinical Practice Guidelines 2019*. Bridgwater: Class Professional Publishing.

McNab, D. et al. (2020). Development and application of 'systems thinking' principles for quality improvement. *BMJ Open Quality* [online]. Available from: https://bmjopenquality.bmj.com/content/9/1/e000714

Meadows, D.H. (2008). *Thinking in Systems: A Primer*. Wright, D. (ed.) Vermont: Chelsea Green Publishing.

Mikolaizak, A.S. et al. (2016). A multidisciplinary intervention to prevent subsequent falls and health service use following fall-related paramedic care: a randomised controlled trial. *Age and Ageing*. 46(2): 200–207.

Moran, C.G. et al. (2018). Changing the system – major trauma patients and their outcomes in the NHS (England) 2008–17. *eClinicalMedicine*. 2: 13–21.

NHS Education for Scotland (2018). Systems Thinking for Everyday Work (STEW) [online]. Available from: https://www.clahrc-gm.nihr.ac.uk/media/Resources/Kidney%20Health/STEW%20Cards%20Final.pdf

Reason, J. (2000). Human error: models and management. *British Medical Journal*. 320: 768–770.

Resuscitation Academy (2018). *10 Steps for Improving Survival from Cardiac Arrest*. 2nd Ed. [online]. Available from: https://www.resuscitationacademy.org/ebook/

Scottish Government (2019). Out-of-Hospital Cardiac Arrest data linkage project: 2017–18 results [online]. Available from: https://www.gov.scot/publications/scottish-out-hospital-cardiac-arrest-data-linkage-project-2017-18-results/

Shorrock, S. (2017). The varieties of human work. *Safety Differently* [online]. Available from: https://www.safetydifferently.com/the-varieties-of-human-work/

Shorrock, S. (2019). Four kinds of thinking: 2. Systems thinking [online]. Available from: https://humanisticsystems.com/2019/11/25/four-kinds-of-thinking-2-systems-thinking/

Snooks, H.A. et al. (2017). Paramedic assessment of older adults after falls, including community care referral pathway: cluster randomised trial. *Annals of Emergency Medicine*. 70(4): 495–505.

The Health Foundation (2010). Evidence scan: Complex adaptive systems [online]. Available from: https://www.health.org.uk/sites/default/files/ComplexAdaptiveSystems.pdf

Wilson, J.R. (2014). Fundamentals of systems ergonomics/human factors. *Applied Ergonomics* [online]. 45(1): 5–13. Available from: https://www.ncbi.nlm.nih.gov/pubmed/23684119

Chapter 5
Human-Centred Design
Shelly Jeffcott

> In this chapter:
> - The power and significance of design in human factors and ergonomics (HF/E)
> - Principles of human-centred design which aim to support humans in the system
> - Barriers to design in healthcare and the opportunities a system focus can bring
> - The three domains of design in HF/E, with examples within a pre-hospital context

Introduction

Historically, in health and social care systems, there has been a focus on how to protect 'safe systems' from the 'unsafe people' working in them. HF/E addresses this myth. It provides a new lens to investigate complexity, alongside a set of approaches that centre around design *for* and *with* people. Design is a crucial tool to help to make systems easier and safer to work in.

A discussed in Chapters 1 and 2, HF/E is a discipline that explores the capabilities, limitations and needs of people in order to drive the design process. It flips things on its head. HF/E recognises the inherent fragility in our systems and the need to harness human-centred design to build strength and safety, with the aim to improve performance and well-being.

Wilson (2014) underlines the central role of design in HF/E. He defines it as 'understanding the interactions between people and all other elements within a system, and design in light of this understanding'. People are the part of our healthcare system that enables us to navigate complexity and create safety, so the aim of HF/E design is to support people in their work. Chapanis (1996) adds that, 'Human factors research discovers and applies information about human behaviour,

Chapter 5 – Human-Centred Design

abilities, limitations, and other characteristics to the design of tools, machines, systems, tasks, and jobs, and environments for productive, safe, comfortable, and effective human use.' HF/E is about fitting work around the human and *not* the other way around. In healthcare, unfortunately, we often set people up to fail and then blame them when they do. Historically, design has been neglected.

Alongside many other commentators, Reason (1990) is keen to move from a model of errant humans in safe systems and believes that 'Rather than being the main instigators of an accident, operators tend to be inheritors of system defects created by poor design, incorrect installation, faulty maintenance and bad management decisions.' The reality is that human beings usually make mistakes because the systems, tasks and products that they work with are not designed to fit their needs and goals.

This chapter will illustrate how design should play a crucial role in supporting quality and safety in our health and social care systems, including pre-hospital care and paramedic practice. It helps to explain some of the cultural reasons why design has been largely overlooked in this sector. The important concept of human-centred design (HCD) is introduced, including how to use this approach to design for and with people. The goal of this chapter is to highlight the power of design and the need to break out of a culture that still focuses on errant workers. We must expect and demand much more to protect our patients and staff.

The Role and Importance of Design

The discipline of design, as it has come to be understood and practised over the past 50 years, can be defined as 'to plan the creation of a product or service with the intention of improving human experience with respect to a specified problem' (Pearsall and Hanks, 2001). In the face of growing systems complexity, design can help us to discover solutions to some of our most challenging problems. Design can lead health and social care away from simple, local fixes to a true systems approach.

As we learnt in Chapter 4, systems thinking is more than a set of tools. It requires a deeper dive into problems, with an appreciation of the whole rather than parts, and a focus on interconnections across all core elements. Many argue that health and social care needs a new focus on design and systems thinking to bring interdisciplinary, human-centred approaches to patient and staff safety.

A seminal Department of Health and Design Council report entitled 'Design for Patient Safety' acknowledged that the use of design in other safety-critical industries had produced significant improvements in the domains of safety, quality and efficiency and recommended that a similar approach be taken within healthcare (Buckle et al, 2003). The report stated that the National Health Service (NHS) was '... seriously out of step with modern thinking and practice with respect to designing for safety, with insufficient grasp of the value and significance of design, and the techniques for managing and implementing design improvements'. It helped to start a whole new dialogue on design in the NHS.

Introduction

Designing with People

The term 'co-design' has become a buzz word to describe a well-established approach to creative practice, particularly in the public sector. Specifically, in health and social care, it is the act of creating ideas for intervention with frontline staff, patients and families so that product or service design both meet their needs and are usable. However, co-design is underutilised, with patient involvement often tokenistic, resulting in missed opportunities for improvement (Sutton et al, 2015).

Participatory ergonomics is an approach taken in HF/E that refers to the active involvement of workers in developing and implementing workplace changes to improve productivity and reduce risks related to safety and health (Burgess-Limerick, 2018). It has been shown to increase comfort and productivity when done successfully (Vink et al, 2006). A participatory or 'co-design' approach is fundamental to being able to use knowledge from staff and patients to improve the design of work.

As introduced in Chapter 4, the Systems Engineering Initiative for Patient Safety (SEIPS) model helps us to think about all the relevant factors within a work system where design or re-design could be tackled to improve positive outcomes. The model draws on three core HF/E principles: systems-orientation, person-centredness, and design-driven improvements (Holden et al, 2013). Systems-orientation refers to taking a holistic approach and studying the healthcare system as a whole. Person-centredness puts people at the heart of healthcare work with the assumption that tools, technologies and support systems must be designed and developed with an understanding of their strengths and limitations. Finally, design-driven improvements focus on improving healthcare work via the development of tools and work activities that can optimise individual, team and organisational performance at all system levels.

The Design of Everyday Things

Effective design can help us deliver systems and products that are intuitive, simple to understand, simple to use and within which it is difficult to make errors. Don Norman wrote a visionary text in the 1980s called 'The Design of Everyday Things'. His philosophy is underpinned by the principle that **'If the system lets you make the error, it is badly designed. And if the system induces you to make the error, then it is *really* badly designed'** (Norman, 1988). He refers to 'design error' as 'when humans fail to meet arbitrary, inhuman requirements of machines', and asks people to consider that when they next fail using a product or service, that it is the design that is at fault. A very simple but radical idea!

Karsh et al (2006) went on to argue that an HF/E approach to designing healthcare delivery systems, which supports professional performance and hazard reduction, will yield significant patient safety benefits. It seems clear that we must make it easier for those working in health and social care systems to provide safe, effective and person-centred care. The tools, tasks, technologies and processes of work need to set people up to succeed as often as possible, so good design is critical.

Chapter 5 – Human-Centred Design

Affordances

Norman (1988) discusses how to make design intuitive and user friendly. He refers to a key concept called an *affordance*. Affordances are the properties of a thing that communicate what it can be used for. We understand a chair affords us to sit on it and a window affords us to look through it.

Norman famously uses the simple example of doors to show that if affordances are ignored, users will make errors and experience discomfort (Figure 5.1). How many times have you tried to push a door open that you should have pulled, and vice versa? When affordances are not considered in design – and even where signage is used to try to combat a mismatch – people may not be able to effectively and reliably use an object. A door plate affords us to push it and a door handle affords us to pull it. A so-called 'Norman door' breaks this convention since, for example, a handle is on a door we are expected to push and not pull open. These doors can be relatively commonplace but a fine example of what happens when affordances are not used to support the user in the design of everyday things.

Natural Mapping

Another design concept highlighted by Norman (1988) is called *natural mapping*. Natural mapping takes advantage of spatial analogies. It is an intuitive association or relationship between two sets of objects, where one can be a controller and the other can be an object which you require to assist your work in some way. So, for example, designers will ensure that the layout of control panels will mirror the equipment being activated or manipulated (Figure 5.2). There are many instances, however, where the controls do not signal what actions are possible and how they should be done.

In the pre-hospital setting, urgency can be a characteristic of patient care, so it is vital that ambulance clinicians have a familiarity and mastery of the equipment they use. A recent report into English Ambulance Trusts, however, showed that most Trusts use different specifications when converting their ambulances and 32 different types were in use (Carter, 2018). This lack of standardisation compounds design issues since ambulance clinicians may be required to know how to use different versions of equipment to perform the same tasks on different shifts. While Norman talks of other ways to use design to support users, affordances and natural mapping are simple and helpful starter concepts to think about.

Design for Patient Safety

Preventable patient harm affects nearly one out of 20 patients in healthcare services (Panagioti et al, 2017). In 2017, 23% of all deaths in the UK were considered avoidable (Office for National Statistics, 2017). As discussed in Chapter 1, limited research exists examining the extent to which patient safety events occur in paramedicine, but an estimated 50–90% of incidents are never reported (Sinclair et al, 2018). Because of this lack of feedback, and often a lack of capacity and capability to analyse the incidents that are reported (Macrae, 2016), the underlying causes of error are not addressed and innovative solutions for lasting safety can be missed.

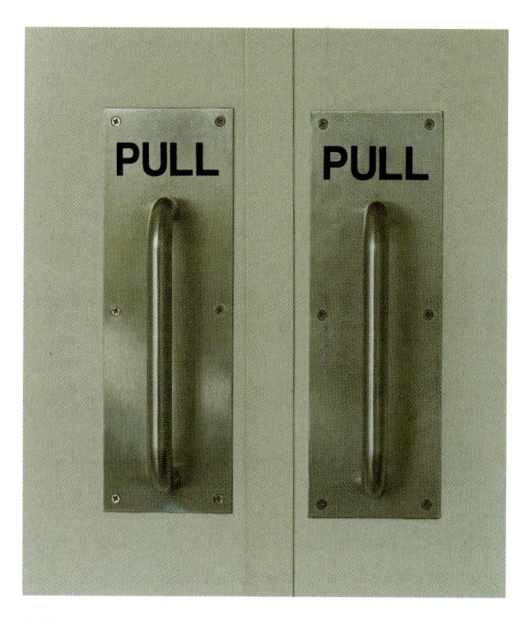

Design for Patient Safety

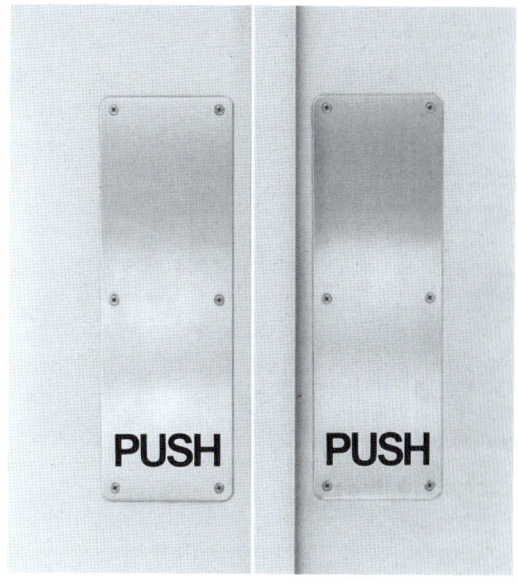

(a)   (b)

Examples of doors which intuitively follow the affordances of a handle (to pull) and a door plate (to push).

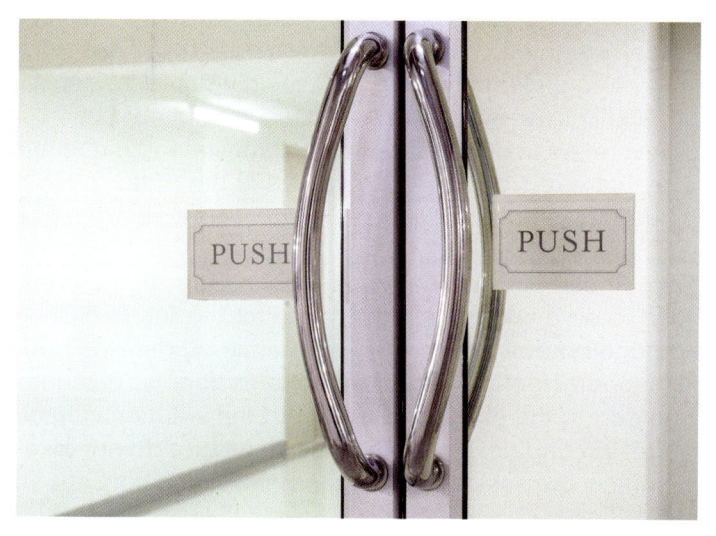

(c) Example of doors which are counter-intuitive to the pull affordance of a handle and force the user to push. The sign to 'push' may help the user not to make an error but commonly this will not override the signal to continue to pull the handle to try to open the door.

Figure 5.1 – Exploring affordances
Source: (a) NENUN/Shutterstock (b) Chulika/Shutterstock (c) nicepix/Shutterstock

Chapter 5 – Human-Centred Design

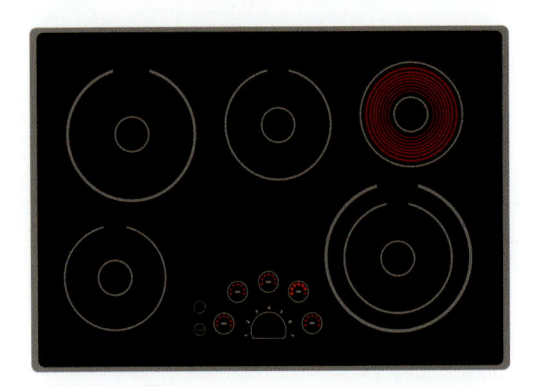

(a) Example of a good natural mapping where the cooker dials match the same layout of the cooker hobs that they control.

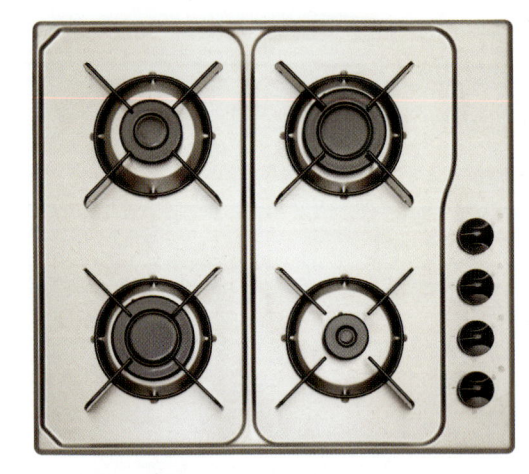

(b) Example of a bad natural mapping where there is ambiguity between the cooker dials and the cooker hobs that they control.

Figure 5.2 – Exploring natural mapping
Source: (a) Constantine Pankin/Shutterstock (b) ppart/Shutterstock

A recent scoping review of patient safety in ambulance services by Fisher et al (2015) concluded, 'Patient safety needs to become a more prominent consideration for ambulance services, rather than operational pressures, including targets and driving the service.' If you asked any frontline member of an ambulance service what their priority is they would likely answer 'to ensure the safety of our patients'. But patient safety in this context refers to an organisational commitment to a reliable system of care delivery so that errors are either prevented or learnt from, and a culture of safety involving healthcare professionals and patients is built.

The procurement and use of equipment and technologies in the pre-hospital settings was found to be a priority research area for the future (Fisher et al, 2015). There is a huge potential to make a difference by thinking about design for patient safety to support frontline ambulance professionals. Technology has been described as both part of the problem and part of the solution in healthcare. This stems from poor design and development processes that do not take account of the needs of humans in the system, leading to unintended consequences (Powell-Cope et al, 2008).

Healthcare is commonly faced with: poor technology design that does not adhere to HF/E principles; poor technology interfaces with the staff, patient or environment; inadequate testing and planning for implementation of a new technology into practice; and inadequate maintenance of technologies through time to ensure safety standards are upheld (IOM, 2004). The pre-hospital arena has a unique set of challenges for practitioners, and providing the best tools for the job is crucial.

A Defibrillator Case Study

Defibrillators are one of the most important pieces of equipment in any ambulance service, and are deployed in a wide variety of settings, such as roads, lounge rooms and the back of the ambulance. This means they are used in all weather, poor lighting conditions and often in a moving vehicle. For pre-hospital use, these devices need to be designed for a specific and complex set of user needs.

The Stryker Physio Control LIFEPAK® 12 and 15 cardiac monitor/defibrillators (see Figure 5.3) are helpful examples of how equipment design can be enhanced, after considering how the operator interacts with it. It was improved to make it easier for the ambulance clinician to do the right thing when using it during critical phases of care, which are likely to be accompanied by high workload, stress and distractions.

The LIFEPAK® 15 is a later model than the LIFEPAK® 12, and some subtle but important changes can be seen in the control panel of the later model. One of the main differences is the shape of the 'shock' button. In the earlier model, the shock button is the same shape as the other buttons around it. In the updated model, the shock button is distinctly different from the other buttons and also has an electricity

| LIFEPAK® 12 defibrillator display panel | LIFEPAK® 15 adapted display panel |

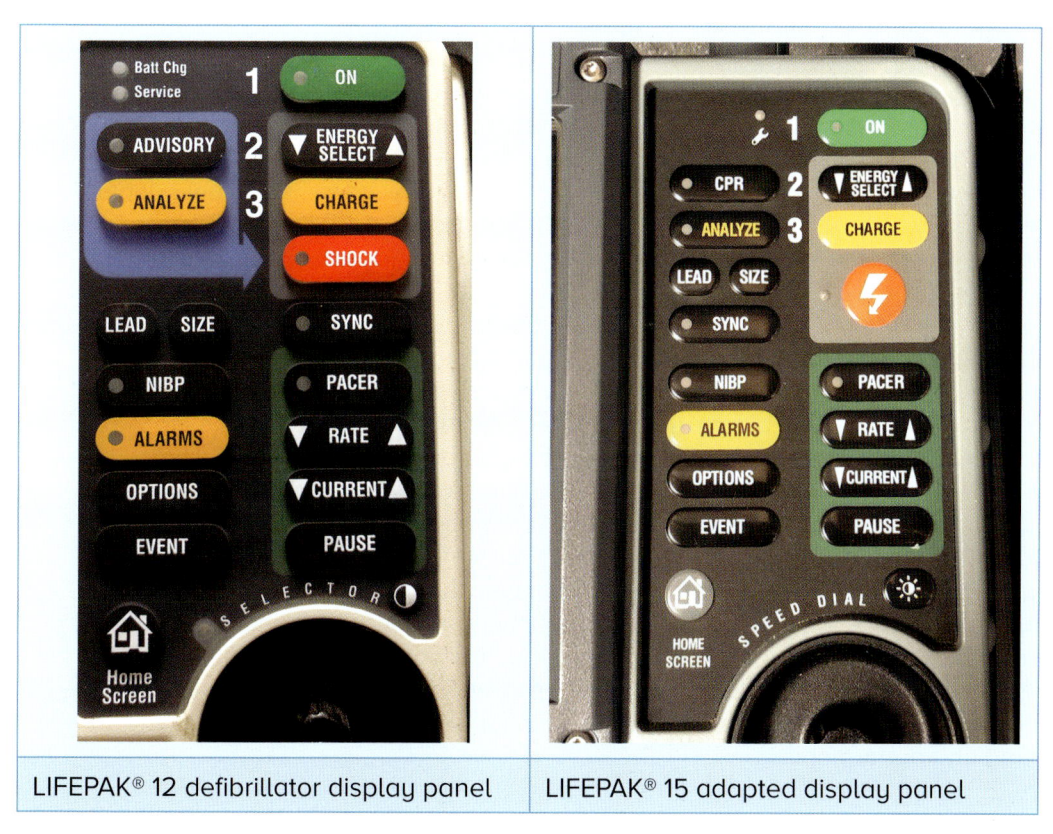

Figure 5.3 – Exploring defibrillator design
Source: © University of Hertfordshire. Reproduced with permission

symbol rather than a word to differentiate it more easily. These enhancements have been made to minimise the likelihood of the wrong button being pressed at the time of shock delivery, reducing potential user confusion with the 'on' button which is nearby and illuminated. That could result in the machine depowering and a delay in defibrillation.

This example shows how design could potentially lead users to make errors. Small changes can make big differences and patient safety can be 'designed into' devices. It is vital to look at incidents with such devices involving different user groups and settings, since the same 'errors' occurring in varying circumstances often indicate deeper problems in the user interface design.

Barriers to Design in Healthcare

'Behavioural-Based Safety'

In healthcare, the response when a frontline professional makes a mistake has historically been to blame and punish (Leape, 1997). Individuals are often viewed as careless and culpable, and most remedial action focuses on them (Dekker, 2006). As a result, a variety of programmes aiming to improve safety by changing the behaviour of workers now exist, referred to as 'behavioural modification' or 'behavioural-based safety' (Ajzen, 1988).

Typically, these interventions involve identifying unsafe versus safe behaviours, setting goals and giving feedback on safety performance which aims to change workers' behaviour (Cooper, 2006). They vary wildly in their effectiveness and, even with positive results, their sustainability is problematic since success is routinely dependent on campaigns and targeted efforts that are often short-lived. It is much rarer to focus instead on how the environment, technology and tools, for example, could have provided more reliable support for safe and effective practice by frontline professional behaviours. Unfortunately, an emphasis on behaviours comes from both management and from individuals themselves and is an embedded, enduring problem.

'When a flower doesn't bloom, you fix the environment in which it grows, not the flower' (Den Heijer, 2018). This quote can also be applied to the situation within healthcare. Why do we focus so much on the flowers, otherwise known as our frontline staff, in lieu of other solutions within the healthcare environment? Design could bring much more widespread, sustainable and positive changes for our workforce and patients. Historically, it seems that a fixation on professional responsibility has propagated the idea that changing people's behaviour is the preferable route to preventing harm. Yet behaviour is the symptom of poorly designed systems. It should only legitimately become a focus after you have successfully managed to implement systems-level interventions to improve well-being and performance.

Person Approach

There needs to be a much greater scrutiny on how we set people up to succeed and make failure difficult. Task and process design, procurement for safety and considering how to optimise environmental conditions to boost human performance and well-being are critical (Karsh et al, 2006). Whatever happens, a move from the person to a systems approach to 'human error' is essential to start asking questions about how and where we can use design better (Wilson, 2014). The person approach to 'human error' is a serious deterrent to learning and improvement. Professor Lucian Leape (1997), a forefather of the modern patient safety movement of the late 1990s, famously stated 'The single greatest impediment to error prevention in the medical industry is that we punish people for making mistakes.'

Punishment and Perfection Myths

The person approach to 'human error' is linked to two myths that we must eradicate if we want to make healthcare systems safer; the punishment myth and the perfection myth (Leape, 2002). The punishment myth relates to the belief that if we punish healthcare professionals who make mistakes, they will be more careful in the future and make fewer errors. The perfection myth is then the belief that if people try hard enough, they will not make errors. How many of us have worked in organisations where we felt the negative impact, through blame and fear, of the person approach to error? It is not isolated to healthcare but it is particularly prevalent in this industry.

Fundamental Attribution Error

Healthcare does not have a monopoly on the punishment and perfection myths. They happen in many other industries and walks of life. An unfortunate focus on individuals, and away from systems design and the wider context, is part of something called the 'fundamental attribution error' (Ross, 1977) and happens in many other industries and walks of life. This is the tendency for people to overemphasise the role of personal characteristics and ignore situational factors when judging others' behaviour. Because of the fundamental attribution error, we tend to believe that others do bad things because they are bad people. This is especially damaging in safety-critical systems as we are less likely to employ design fixes and to stop others from making the same error. The fundamental attribution error can lead to explanations staying simple and punitive in nature.

'Make Do and Mend'

'Make do and mend' is an expression born from the austerity of World War II in the UK. It was a central mindsight that helped to encourage and support both recycling and extending the lifetime of goods and consumables (Ministry of Information, 2007).

Our healthcare systems are under huge amounts of strain in terms of matching limited resources with ever-growing demand, particularly from an ageing demographic in westernised countries. People are living much longer than they did in the past, many surviving into their 90s, often with complex multi-morbidities. There is a large emphasis now on how to reorganise in order to get more from what we have. Yet, the common perception by those at the coalface is that finances drive decisions and the expectation is for them to keep delivering more with less (Robertson et al, 2017). This puts a huge strain on staff, and the idea of 'make do and mend' – in terms of the equipment, technologies and all 'the kit' that staff use daily to do their jobs – is increasingly relevant in the context of a modern, struggling healthcare system.

Chapter 5 – Human-Centred Design

Many frontline staff, and middle managers alike, have become resigned and do not submit requests for different or better equipment to help improve performance and well-being. They know how restrictive budgets are and that there is unlikely to be changes to the technologies that they come to rely on, especially if these changes require greater expenditure. Invariably people shrug their shoulders and accept the status quo. We rarely challenge the procurement process or decisions that are made, which are arguably driven by cost and safety, but not usability (Buckle et al, 2003).

'Normalisation of Deviance'

In her analysis of the Challenger disaster, Diane Vaughan (1996) described an organisational/social phenomenon called 'normalisation of deviance'. This occurs when small, incremental erosions to safety and quality over time became the norm. In the context of this growing 'make do and mend' culture, a similar normalisation of deviance is occurring with this passive acceptance of putting up with and not challenging the design of the environment, technology and processes around us.

It is the antithesis of the HF/E discipline and tradition, to allow human operators to be crammed into ill-fitting systems, producing higher levels of preventable harm and short-sighted attempts at interventions. According to Zhang (2005), 'In healthcare, the culture is still to train people to adapt to poorly designed technology, rather than to design technology to fit people's characteristics.' We need to begin to break out of a tradition which looks to change people first.

'Good Provider Fallacy'

People who go into caring professions commonly fit into something called the 'good provider fallacy', which, put simply, is about going the extra mile for patients and not giving up, despite obstacles and error traps (Henriksen and Dayton, 2006). It is making things work, even if they don't work for you! Frontline clinicians can almost universally be described as having an impeccable work ethic, commitment and compassion. Henriksen et al (2008) state that 'Many, no doubt, take pride in their individual competence, resourcefulness, and ability to solve problems on the run during the daily processes of care.' But this compounds the problem of systems not designed to support frontline professionals in their safety-critical roles.

Tucker and Edmondson (2003) conducted a study of hospital work process failures (for example, missing supplies, malfunctioning equipment, incomplete/inaccurate information, unavailable personnel). They found that the failures elicited work-arounds and quick fixes by nurses 93% of the time, and subsequent reports of the failure to someone who could do something about it only 7% of the time. While this strategy for problem-solving satisfies the immediate patient care need, from a systems perspective it means that the multitude of contributing factors and opportunities to address design issues to prevent re-occurrences – and improve the working lives of staff – remain unresolved. It is often the case that frontline staff do not report concerns about their working environment and equipment because they believe that there is futility in expecting change in these areas (Macrae, 2016). We need to create a new culture which encourages openness when talking about how design may be letting us down. Critical to this, is having organisations who understand the role of design in both safety and quality of care.

Design Focusing on People

User-Centred Design

The aim of the user-centred design process is to ensure that the design of a product or service remains focused upon who will use it, in what context, and with what aim. Historically it was an approach used to combat design methods that were typically led by technology, where businesses would find ways to use technology to solve a problem and then focus on features and functionality to create a product. Users were an afterthought, so when the product launched, its users were expected and required to adapt to the technology. The philosophy behind user-centred design proposes that the product or service should instead adapt to the user.

Norman and Draper (1986) first described the concept: '… user-centred design emphasizes that the purpose of the system is to serve the user, not to use a specific technology, not to be an elegant piece of programming. The needs of the users should dominate the design of the interface, and the needs of the interface should dominate the design of the rest of the system.' This means that any design process should start with a full understanding of user requirements to help them to achieve their goals which, in a healthcare context is, safe, effective and person-centred care (Henriksen et al, 2008).

To understand what users want and need, it is crucial to not only ask them questions but also to observe them at work, as they use technologies and equipment to complete daily tasks. In this way it is possible to tap into 'work-as-done', not just 'work-as-imagined', and to understand what the user experience is really like when things go right and wrong (Shorrock and Williams, 2016). As discussed in Chapter 4, 'work-as-imagined' (WAI) is what is formally mandated in policies and procedures as the way that work *should* happen. 'Work-as-done' (WAD) is then the real process by which people get their work done. The gap between WAI and WAD often represents the ill-fitting design of systems to support workers. WAD reflects natural variability in systems and multiple adaptations that staff must routinely make (EUROCONTROL, 2017).

Human-Centred Design

User-centred design is a subset of human-centred design since not everyone can be categorised as a 'user', but good design must take account of human needs and capabilities. Humans, in complex systems like healthcare, should be central to the process of design, and developing and testing solutions. They should also ultimately reap benefits from products and services that work for them and make their work, in the form of interactions, as easy as possible.

Norman (2008) notes, 'The whole point of human-centred design is to tame complexity, to turn what would appear to be a complicated tool into one that fits the task, that is understandable, usable, enjoyable.' Designing for users has turned into designing for people and HF/E is key to both.

Chapter 5 – Human-Centred Design

Signage

As part of his thesis on what constitutes good or bad design, Norman (1988) reminds us that when objects or technologies require signage to support and guide human use, it is often a big clue to us that the design is not intuitive, and/or does not fit our mental models or expectations of its activities. 'Any time you see signs or labels added to a device, it is an indication of bad design: a simple lock should not require instructions.' In contrast, 'good design is actually a lot harder to notice than poor design, in part because good design fits our needs so well the design is invisible' (Norman, 1988). Figure 5.4(a) demonstrates a poor design with complicated signage to try to compensate and guide the user not to make an error, in contrast with (b) a good, intuitive design that has only simple instruction for the user.

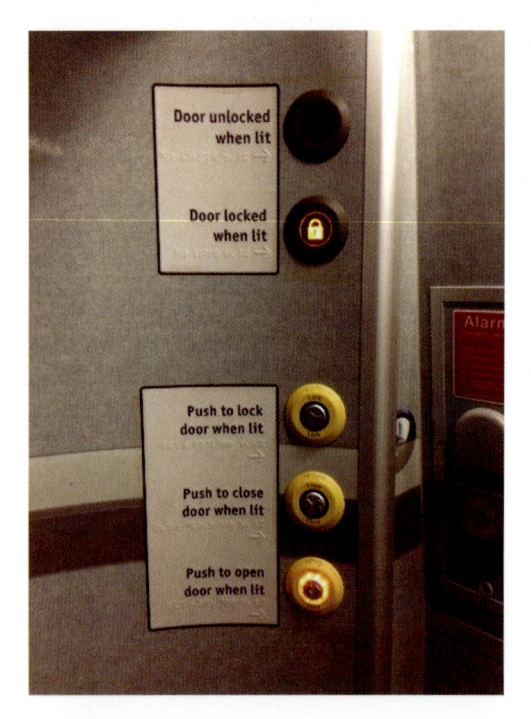

(a) Example of complicated signage to guide a user to understand how to close, lock and open a train toilet door. The number of instructions required for this simple operation is disproportionate and may reflect where the design is lacking. Anxiety created by these complex door locking arrangements can cause passengers to avoid using toilets on trains and wait until they alight to use station toilets.

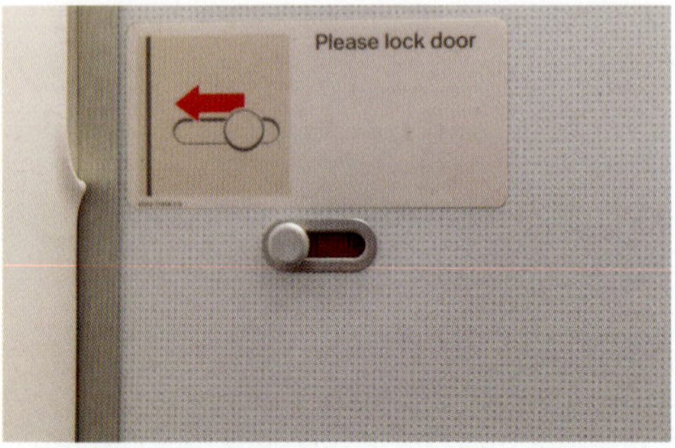

(b) Example of an aeroplane toilet door lock, with its dual funtionality which means that sliding the door lock to secure the door while using the toilet will also turn the light in the toilet cubicle on. Some aeroplane models have a lock symbol, like this one, with a directional arrow indicating which way to slide the lock, but often there is no need for any signage to assist users.

Figure 5.4 – Exploring signage in design
Source: (a) Gary Rutherford (b) Shutterstock/jannoon028

Design Focusing on People

Human-Centred Design for Interactive Systems

Best practice in HF/E ensures human-centred design processes are adopted to understand, specify and accommodate the needs of people working in complex systems. Human-centred design (HCD) is defined in an HF/E context as '... an approach to interactive systems development that aims to make systems usable and useful by focusing on the users, their needs and requirements, and by applying HF/E, and usability knowledge and techniques' (ISO, 2019).

ISO stands for the 'International Organization for Standardization' – the world's largest developer and publisher of voluntary International Standards.

These ISO Standards ensure that all products and services are safe for use and are reliable and of sound quality. Following ISO allows organisations to limit errors, support users, reduce costs and minimise waste, increasing productivity.

ISO 9241, Part 210 is called 'Human-centred design for interactive systems'. It provides an HCD approach that follows several fundamental principles (ISO, 2019):

- design based on an explicit understanding of users, tasks and environments
- involving users throughout design and development
- making sure the process is iterative and informed by user-centred evaluation
- addressing the whole user experience and drawing from multidisciplinary experience.

The many reported benefits of taking an HCD approach (Giacomin, 2014) include:

- increasing the productivity of users by making things easier to understand and use
- improving the user experience by addressing usability and accessibility issues
- reducing discomfort and stress and the likelihood of harm events.

Bias and Mayhew (1994) strongly advocate the integration of HCD from the very start of the design life cycle, i.e. the requirements phase, since it creates a greater number of design alternatives and can eliminate the cost, in the later deployment phase, of needing to re-work and make changes because elements of the design were not fully scoped or tested appropriately. It is critical to involve HF/E expertise as early as possible to help investigate and define user requirements and test changes.

ISO 9241, Part 210: 'Dialogue Principles'

An important part of helping guide people's use of ISO 9241-210 and to support HCD are the 'dialogue principles'. This is unusual terminology for a set of usability heuristics (or 'rules of thumb') that apply to the interaction of people and information systems. The ISO standard refers to this interaction as a 'dialogue' and describes the 'dialogue principles' as a framework for applying HF/E in healthcare design.

Chapter 5 – Human-Centred Design

The seven principles, with accompanying questions to ask yourself, are (ISO, 2019):

1. *suitability for the task* (does it suit the user's task and skill level?)
2. *self-descriptiveness* (does it make it clear what's going on and what the user should do next?)
3. *controllability* (is the user in control of the interaction?)
4. *conformity with user expectations* (does it conform with user expectations?)
5. *error tolerance* (is it forgiving of errors?)
6. *suitability for individualisation* (can interaction and presentation be customised to suit the user?)
7. *suitability for learning* (does it support learning?)

Usability

Usability is an important concept when thinking about design since it is '... the ease of use and acceptability of a system for a specific class of users carrying out particular tasks in a specific environment' (Holzinger, 1995). Usability is defined by the following five quality components: learnability, efficiency, memorability, error recovery and satisfaction (Nielsen, 1994).

Unfortunately, usability is traditionally left out of procurement processes, which commonly evaluate the utility of the device (i.e. can the device perform the required functions?) and the financial feasibility (i.e. pricing options and competitive bids) but often does not extend to user experience or usability testing (Namshirin et al, 2011).

An expert commentator in the area of human–computer interaction and usability, Ben Shneiderman (2002), notes 'The old computing was about what computers could do; the new computing is about what users can do. Successful technologies are those that are in harmony with users' needs. They must support relationships and activities that enrich the users' experiences.' This should be a given and not a luxury in healthcare, particularly in pre-hospital settings where every second counts.

Procurement

When usability is not given equal emphasis with utility and financial feasibility in procurement decisions, there is an increased probability of patients suffering harm or close calls (Davies et al, 2007). Conversely, procurement based on usability has the potential to tackle preventable harm (Namshirin et al, 2011).

It has been shown that safety and performance benefits of incorporating HF/E evaluations into procurement activities include: improved user performance (fewer user errors and high user satisfaction), fewer implementation problems, increased local improvement opportunities to support local use, and improved end-user readiness for change (Lin et al, 1998; Davies et al, 2007; Namshirin et al, 2011).

HF/E Evaluation Methods

Four HF/E evaluation methods for exploring usability in procurement decisions are:

1. *Usability walkthrough*, which is an informal usability inspection method that involves end-users exploring and interacting with a medical device, equipment or technology and commenting on their experiences to an evaluator (Bias, 1994).

2. *Heuristic evaluation*, which is a usability inspection method that involves HF/E experts assessing the design of a medical device, equipment or technology against established usability principles (Nielsen, 1994; ISO, 2019). A good heuristic evaluation requires at least 3–5 evaluators who work independently, and then compare and combine results. This should lead to a list of potential usability issues which are usually ranked in the order of their severity.

3. *Usability testing*, which is systematic observation of a representative sample of end-users completing realistic task scenarios with a medical device, equipment or technology (Dumas and Redish, 1999) often, but not always, outside of their work environment. This usually happens in a simulated way. In a pre-hospital setting, possible systems for usability testing may include, for example, defibrillators, medicines, electronic patient records.

4. *Field study*, which is about observation and/or feedback from end-users who use a medical device, equipment or technology for a defined period of time, in order to observe enough variation in different scenarios, in clinical practice (Israelski, 2010).

Design Domains in HF/E

Design of any complex system calls for careful decisions affecting the demands placed on human perceptual, cognitive and motor systems, in addition to the organisational context (Helander, 2006). There are three distinct domains to explore the implications of design in HF/E and each is outlined below, in relation to some examples pertinent to the pre-hospital setting. This is to start you thinking about ways in which design and patient safety could be improved in your work setting.

Physical HF/E

Physical HF/E examines the topics of human anatomy, anthropometrics, physiology and biomechanics in relation to the interactions of the user and the equipment used.

Practical applications of these considerations include workplace layout, working postures, materials handling, repetitive movements and work-related musculoskeletal disorder analysis (Chadwick and Jeffcott, 2013).

The objectives that might be considered in *Physical HF/E design* are to minimise perception time, decision time and manipulation time; to reduce or mitigate the need for excessive physical exertion; and to optimise opportunities for physical movement to promote fitness and well-being.

Chapter 5 – Human-Centred Design

Pre-Hospital Examples

Until very recently, individual vehicle specifications existed for NHS Ambulance Trusts. Although work has begun to standardise the design of emergency ambulances, the unfortunate legacy is that ambulance clinicians may be expected to work with many different ambulance interior layouts, in terms of the location of equipment and consumables. This could impact on both efficiency and safety.

HF/E work evaluating ambulance loading systems, as well as vehicle and equipment risks, helped provide an evidence base for design recommendations to form a new ambulance specification. This has included: access/egress, space and layout, securing people and equipment in transit, communication, security, violence and aggression, hygiene, vehicle engineering and patient experience (Hignett et al, 2009). This will help to address the issue of multiple layouts and unwarranted variation highlighted in the Carter report (2018).

HF/E projects involve direct observation of frontline clinicians in order to understand where physical design could harm either staff or patients and could cause waste in both human and financial terms. Ferreira and Hignett (2005) observed paramedics over 16 shifts (130 hours) carrying out a range of clinical tasks, during a review of the layout of the most common patient compartment in UK ambulances.

The most frequently occurring clinical tasks were checking blood oxygen saturation, oxygen administration, monitoring the heart and checking blood pressure. Access to the equipment and consumables to support these tasks had been designed for the attendant seat (head end of the stretcher). However, their analysis found that paramedics preferred to sit alongside the stretcher which resulted in increased reach distances. The highest frequency tasks were found to include working postures requiring corrective measures over 40% of the time, potentially resulting in injury over long-term exposure (Ferreira and Hignett, 2005).

It is vital to keep today's paramedic workforce healthy, both physically and mentally to optimise their well-being (see Chapter 7). If we don't look after staff, they can't look after patients to the best of their ability. Burnout in health professionals is at an all-time high and positively correlates with poor patient outcomes (Hall et al, 2016). Poor morale in paramedics results from burnout, work overload and poor health (Nirel et al, 2008). However, better design specifications and/or simple modifications can reduce workload and physical stress on their bodies.

Cognitive HF/E

Cognitive HF/E analyses the cognitive processes that affect the user and interactions of the user and technology during task completion. These cognitive processes include memory, reasoning, perception and motor response (see Chapters 8 and 9).

Practical applications of cognitive HF/E include the assessment of human reliability and 'human error', human–computer interaction, mental workload, decision making, skilled performance, work stress and training (Chadwick and Jeffcott, 2013).

The objectives that might be considered in *Cognitive HF/E design* are to ensure consistency of interface design; to ensure a match between technology and the user's mental model; to minimise cognitive load; to allow for error detection and recovery; and to provide feedback to users in the interaction.

Pre-Hospital Examples

There are many tools created in the pre-hospital environment which are designed to reduce the occurrence of errors and support best practice and patient safety. These include (in a non-exhaustive list) standard operating procedures, routine checklists, emergency action checklists, procedural aide-memoires, clinical guidelines and patient safety or equipment alerts.

All these items include prompts designed to help users complete a task or series of tasks and could be grouped together and described as 'cognitive aids'. Although most cognitive aids in healthcare emerge through well-intentioned activity to support teams and individuals, they rarely follow HCD principles in order to support cognition, particularly in emergencies (Marshall, 2013).

Evidence from the HF/E literature suggests that poorly designed cognitive aids may lead to 'unintended consequences', that is, outcomes that are not the ones foreseen and intended by a purposeful action. It is unfortunate to think that tools created to boost patient safety may fail to do so and, worse still, could lead to preventable harm if there is no consideration of the cognitive capabilities and workflow of clinicians during their design (Lintern and Motavalli, 2018).

The intention of cognitive aids is to relieve pressure on memory and attention, particularly in the limited cognitive 'bandwidth' scenarios that characterise paramedic practice. They aim to support better decision making, and team and individual performance to achieve safer outcomes. Cognitive aids used in emergency situations are different from those used in routine settings because of the requirement of the content to be physically and cognitively accessible during times of stress (Kontogiannis, 1996). This makes the argument for good cognitive design even greater in the pre-hospital setting where there can be limited information, time urgency and high acuity patients.

The focus during the development of most cognitive aids is on the accuracy of the technical content, which is based on established guidelines most of the time. In contrast, the presentation of the information and the resultant usability of cognitive aids to support decision making have been less thoroughly considered. Marshall (2013), in his review of cognitive aids during emergencies, found only one that was developed with a systematic design process. Evans et al (2015) adapted an aviation 'Checklist Assessment Tool' into a healthcare context to improve the usability of medical emergency guidelines, but overall there is a lack of HF/E guidance to support the development and use of cognitive aids in health and social care settings (Marshall, 2017).

Chapter 5 – Human-Centred Design

Organisational HF/E

Organisational HF/E seeks to account for the complex interactions within socio-technical systems. It focuses on holistic work system analysis and design by examining the factors that influence stakeholders' work practices, i.e. personnel, technology, environment, tasks and work culture. Subgroups within these categories include teamwork, safety culture, supervision, shift work, scheduling and job satisfaction (Chadwick and Jeffcott, 2013).

The objectives that might be considered in *Organisational HF/E design* are to provide opportunities to workers to learn and develop new skills; to allow worker control over work systems; to support worker access to social support; and to involve users in system design and testing of interventions.

Pre-Hospital Examples

Organisational design is arguably the most neglected of the three types of HF/E design but has significant links to safety (Bourrier, 2005). Rules and organisational routines can be frequently overlooked but have strong impacts on the well-being of workers (Arches, 1991). West (2001) adds 'We all need to become much more conscious of how the way we work together, and the way that care is organised, affects patients' experience of the healthcare system'. Traditionally, ambulance services have a centralised structure, which means most decisions are taken by senior management with layers of hierarchy that are rigid and strictly adhered to in terms of who can 'speak out' (Edmondson, 1999). Progress has been made but there is still a steep power gradient, in many cases, with the challenging of norms not widely supported.

Organisational processes, such as human resource (HR) management practices and procedures, conflict resolution and how incidents and complaints are dealt with, are also important. In this category the literature stresses the relationship between participation in decision making, sense of involvement in the organisation and sense of autonomy and control (Woods and Shattuck, 2000). The role of HR in disciplinary activities after incidents can reinforce a person approach and block learning on how to prevent similar systems failures in future (Dekker, 2006; Macrae, 2016).

There is a lower power gradient and 'just culture' (Reason, 1997) in the multidisciplinary and inter-organisational teams within which many paramedics work in other situations but, overall, a lack of input to the design of interventions and a fear of career-limiting activities (for example, challenging authority, breaking rules that don't fit work) can restrict individuals and impact on patient safety.

A relevant case study in organisational design comes from Mersey Care NHS Foundation Trust, who implemented just culture principles that involved a number of organisational changes. These had corresponding, and overwhelmingly positive, influences on the well-being of individuals, on patient safety and also on performance (Dekker and Breakey, 2016). A reduction in suspensions and dismissals, an increase in the reporting of adverse events, an increase in the number of staff seeking employee assistance, with a reduction in absence due to illness and a decrease in turnover were all reported (Kaur et al, 2019). Organisational design profoundly effects prevailing culture since it dictates and reflects on the ability of staff to do their best work.

Summary

The patient safety movement has made slow progress in the last 25 years. Many have attributed this to a lack of HF/E-based design, leaving interventions that are superficial and gains which cannot be sustained (Braithwaite et al, 2015). Bob Wears, Professor of Emergency Medicine and a strong advocate for HF/E, stated that in healthcare systems 'despite spouting a great deal of rhetoric about systems and "systems thinking" … favoured interventions focus not on systems of care, but rather on restricting and controlling the individuals providing it' (Wears, 2017). It is unfortunate that the patient safety movement has not yet fully appreciated the benefits of human-centred and rapid-prototyping design approaches, instead allowing top-down design mandates to spread without proper testing or user input.

This chapter has outlined just how vital design is for patient and staff safety. We must consider the physical, cognitive and organisational domains of HF/E and promote greater scrutiny of design which impacts our working conditions. We must challenge the mindsets that continue to reinforce a person over a systems approach. A greater push to involve usability testing and incorporating these results into procurement decisions could help staff to have the best tools for the job. The overall objective is to fit the healthcare system to those delivering and receiving care, rather than the other way around, and to stop tolerating preventable harm.

Examples from the pre-hospital setting help illustrate key arguments and provide insights which may inspire you to think more about design and how you could, for instance, start using simple heuristics to examine equipment that you use at work (Nielsen, 1994; ISO, 2019). You may even begin to see with fresh eyes and have new ideas for change. Confusing user interfaces, with mismatches between interface design and actual care requirements or inflexible and non-intuitive systems, all bring significant risk to healthcare tools and technologies which human-centred design can limit. Huge opportunities will arise if we embark on designing with people at the heart and centre. This requires multidisciplinary design teams, with support at all system levels, to listen and learn from each other and from patients and families.

References

Ajzen, I. (1988). *Attitudes, Personality, and Behavior*. Buckingham: Open University Press.

Arches, J. (1991). Social structure, burnout, and job satisfaction. *Social Work*. 36(3): 202–206.

Bias, R. (1994). The pluralistic usability walkthrough: coordinated empathies. In: Nielsen, J., Mack, R. (eds). *Usability Inspection Methods*. New York: John Wiley and Sons.

Bias, R., Mayhew, D. (eds) (1994). *Cost–Justifying Usability*. Burlington, MA: Morgan Kaufmann Publishers.

Bourrier M. (2005). The contribution of organizational design to safety. *European Management Journal*. 23(1): 98–104.

Chapter 5 – Human-Centred Design

Braithwaite, J., Wears, R., Hollnagel, E. (2015). Resilient health care: turning patient safety on its head. *International Journal for Quality in Health Care*. 27(5): 418–420.

Buckle, P. et al. (2003). *Design for Patient Safety: A system-wide design-led approach to tackling patient safety in the NHS*. London: Department of Health Publications.

Burgess-Limerick, R. (2018). Participatory ergonomics: evidence and implementation lessons. *Applied Ergonomics*. 68: 289–293.

Carter, P.R. (2018). Operational productivity and performance in English NHS Ambulance Trusts: unwarranted variations. Official government commissioned review [online]. https://improvement.nhs.uk/documents/3271/Operational_productivity_and_performance_NHS_Ambulance_Trusts_final.pdf

Chadwick, L., Jeffcott, S. (2013). A brief introduction to human factors engineering. *Transfusion*. 53(6): 1166–1167.

Chapanis, A. (1996). *Human Factors in Systems Engineering*. New York: Wiley & Sons.

Cooper, D. (2006). Exploratory analyses of the effects of managerial support and feedback consequences on behavioral safety maintenance. *Journal of Organizational Behavior Management*. 26: 1–41.

Davies, J., Caird, J., Chisholm, S. (2007). Trying before buying: human factors evaluations of new medical technology. In: Anca, J. (ed.). *Multimodal Safety Management and Human Factors: Crossing the borders of medical, aviation, road and rail industries*. Aldershot: Ashgate, pp. 316–323.

Dekker, S. (2006). *The Field Guide to Understanding Human Error*. Aldershot: Ashgate.

Dekker, S.W., Breakey, H. (2016). 'Just culture': Improving safety by achieving substantive, procedural and restorative justice. *Safety Science*. 85: 187–193.

Den Heijer, A. (2018). *Nothing You Don't Already Know: Remarkable reminders about meaning, purpose, and self-realization* [e-book]. Amazon online publishing.

Dul, J. et al. (2012). A strategy for human factors/ergonomics: developing the discipline and profession. *Ergonomics*. 55: 377–395.

Dumas, J., Redish, J. (1999). *A Practical Guide to Usability Testing*. Revised Ed. Portland, OR: Intellect Books.

Edmondson, A. (1999). Psychological safety and learning behavior in work teams. *Administrative Science Quarterly*. 44(2): 350–383.

EUROCONTROL (2017). Work-as-Imagined & Work-as-Done. *HindSight*. 25, Summer. Brussels: EUROCONTROL.

Evans, D. et al. (2015). Cognitive Aids in Medicine Assessment Tool (CMAT): preliminary validation of a novel tool for the assessment of emergency cognitive aids. *Anaesthesia*. 70(8): 922–932.

Ferreira, J., Hignett, S. (2005). Reviewing ambulance design for clinical efficiency and paramedic safety. *Applied Ergonomics*. 36(1): 97–105.

Fisher, J. et al. (2015). Patient Safety in Ambulance Services: A scoping review. *Health Services and Delivery Research*. 3(21).

Giacomin, J. (2014). What is human centred design? *The Design Journal*. 17(4): 606–623.

Hall, L. et al. (2016). Healthcare staff wellbeing, burnout, and patient safety: a systematic review. *PLOS One*. 11(7): 1–12.

Helander, M. (2006). *A Guide to Human Factors and Ergonomics*. 2nd Ed. Boca Raton: CRC Press.

Henriksen, K., Dayton, E. (2006). Organizational silence and hidden threats to patient safety. *Health Services Research*. 41(4, part 2): 1539–1554.

Henriksen, K. et al. (2008). Understanding adverse events: a human factors framework. In: Hughes, R. (ed.). *Patient Safety and Quality: An evidence-based handbook for nurses*. Rockville, MD: Agency for Healthcare Research and Quality (US), Chapter 5.

References

Hignett, S., Crumpton, E., Coleman, R. (2009). Designing emergency ambulances for the 21st century. *Emergency Medicine Journal*. 26(2): 135–40.

Holden, R.J. et al. (2013). SEIPS 2.0: A human factors framework for studying and improving the work of healthcare professionals and patients. *Ergonomics*. 56(11): 1669–1686.

Holzinger, A. (1995). Usability engineering methods for software developers. *Communications of the ACM*. 48(1): 71–74.

Institute of Medicine (IOM) (2004). *Keeping Patients Safe: Transforming the work environment of nurses*. Washington, D.C.: The National Academies Press.

International Organization for Standardization (ISO) (2019). International Standard ISO 9241-210:2019. Ergonomics of human-system interaction – Part 210: Human-centred design for interactive systems. First Edition. Reference number ISO 9241-210:2010(E), Switzerland. Available from: https://www.iso.org/obp/ui/#iso:std:iso:9241:-210:ed-2:v1:en

Israelski, E. (2010). Testing and evaluation. In: Weinger, M.B., Wiklund, M.E., Gardner-Bonneau, D.J. (eds). *Handbook of Human Factors in Medical Device Design*. Boca Raton: CRC Press.

Karsh, B. et al. (2006). A human factors engineering paradigm for patient safety: designing to support the performance of the healthcare professional. *Quality & Safety in Health Care*. 15(Suppl 1): i59–i65.

Kaur, M. et al. (2019). Restorative just culture: a study of the practical and economic effects of implementing restorative justice in an NHS trust. *MATEC Web of Conferences*. 273, 01007.

Kontogiannis, T. (1996). Stress and operator decision making in coping with emergencies. *International Journal of Human Computer Studies*. 45(1): 75–104.

Leape, L.L. (1997). A systems analysis approach to medical error. *Journal of Evaluation in Clinical Practice*. 3(3): 213–222.

Leape, L. (2002). Striving for perfection. *Clinical Chemistry*. 48(11): 1871–1872.

Lin, L. et al. (1998). Applying human factors to the design of medical equipment: patient-controlled analgesia. *Journal of Clinical Monitoring and Computing*. 14(4): 253–263.

Lintern, G., Motavalli, A. (2018). Healthcare information systems: the cognitive challenge. *BMC Medical Informatics and Decision Making*. 18(3): 1–10.

Macrae, C. (2016). The problem with incident reporting. *BMJ Quality & Safety*. 25: 71–75.

Marshall, S. (2013). The use of cognitive aids during emergencies in anesthesia: a review of the literature. *Anesthesia and Analgesia*. 117(5): 1162–1171.

Marshall, S. (2017). Helping experts and expert teams perform under duress: an agenda for cognitive aid research. *Anaesthesia*. 72(3): 289–295.

Ministry of Information (2007). *Make Do and Mend* (Historic Booklet Series). London: Sabrestorm Publishing.

Namshirin, P., Ibey, A., Lamsdale, A. (2011). Applying a multidisciplinary approach to the selection, evaluation, and acquisition of smart infusion pumps. *Journal of Medical and Biological Engineering*. 31(2): 93–98.

Nielsen, J. (1994). Heuristic evaluation. In: Nielsen, J., Mack, R. (eds). *Usability Inspection Methods*. New York: John Wiley and Sons.

Nirel, N. et al. (2008). Stress, work overload, burnout, and satisfaction among paramedics in Israel. *Prehospital and Disaster Medicine*. 23(6): 537–546.

Norman, D. (1986). Cognitive engineering. In: Norman, D., Draper, S. (eds). *User Centred Systems Design*. Hillsdale, NJ: Lawrence Erlbaum Associates Inc.

Norman, D. (1988). *The Design of Everyday Things*. New York: Basic Books.

Norman, D. (2008). The way I see it - Simplicity is not the answer. *Interactions*. 15(5): 45–46.

Chapter 5 – Human-Centred Design

Norman, D., Draper, S. (eds). (1986). *User Centred Systems Design*. Hillsdale, NJ: Lawrence Erlbaum Associates Inc.

Office for National Statistics (2017). *Avoidable Mortality in the UK: 2017*. Statistical Bulletin Series. Released: 22 February 2019.

Panagioti, M. et al. (2017). Preventable patient harm across health care services: A systematic review and meta-analysis (understanding harmful care). A report for the General Medical Council, UK. Available from: https://www.gmc-uk.org/-/media/documents/preventable-patient-harm-across-health-care-services_pdf-73538295.pdf.

Pearsall, J., Hanks, P. (2001). *The New Oxford Dictionary of English*. Oxford: Oxford University Press.

Powell-Cope, G., Nelson, A., Patterson, E. (2008). Patient care technology and safety. In: Hughes, R. (ed.). *Patient Safety and Quality: An evidence-based handbook for nurses*. Rockville, MD: Agency for Healthcare Research and Quality, Chapter 50.

Reason, J. (1990). *Human Error*. Cambridge: Cambridge University Press.

Reason, J. (1997). *Managing the Risks of Organizational Accidents*. Aldershot: Ashgate.

Robertson, R. et al. (2017). Understanding NHS financial pressures: how are they affecting patient care? The King's Fund, UK. Available from: https://www.kingsfund.org.uk/publications/understanding-nhs-financial-pressures.

Ross, L. (1977). The intuitive psychologist and his shortcomings: distortions in the attribution process. In: *Advances in Experimental Social Psychology* (Vol. 10). New York: Academic Press.

Shneiderman, B. (2002). *Leonardo's Laptop: Human Needs and the New Computing Technologies*. Cambridge, MA: MIT Press.

Shorrock, S., Williams, C. (2016). *Human Factors and Ergonomics in Practice: Improving system performance and human well-being in the real world*. Abingdon-on-Thames: Routledge.

Sinclair, J. et al. (2018). Barriers to self-reporting patient safety incidents by paramedics: a mixed methods study. *Prehospital Emergency Care*. 22: 1–11.

Sutton, E., Eborall, H., Martin, G. (2015). Patient involvement in patient safety: current experiences, insights from the wider literature, promising opportunities? *Public Management Review*. 17: 72–89.

Tucker, A., Edmondson, A. (2003). Why hospitals don't learn from failures: organizational and psychological dynamics that inhibit system change. *Californian Management Review*. 45: 55–72.

Vaughan, D. (1996). *The Challenger Launch Decision – Risky technology, culture, and deviance at NASA*. Chicago, IL: The University of Chicago Press.

Vink, E., Koningsveld, E., Molenbroek, J. (2006). Positive outcomes of participatory ergonomics in terms of greater comfort and higher productivity. *Applied Ergonomics*. 37: 537–546.

Wears, R. (2017). Design: a neglected modality for improvement. *Annals of Emergency Medicine*. 69(3): 315–317.

West, E. (2001). Management matters: the link between hospital organisation and quality of patient care. Quality in Health Care. 10: 40–48.

Wilson, J. (2014). Fundamentals of systems ergonomics/human factors. *Applied Ergonomics*. 45(1): 5–13.

Woods, D., Shattuck, L. (2000). Distant supervision – local action given the potential for surprise. *Cognition, Technology & Work*. 2(4): 242–245.

Zhang, J. (2005). Human-centered computing in health information systems. Part 1: analysis and design. *Journal of Biomedical Informatics*. 38(1): 1–3.

Ziewacz, J. et al. (2011). Crisis checklists for the operating room: development and pilot testing. *Journal of the American College of Surgeons*. 213: 212–217.

Chapter 6
The Patient: An Element of the System

Gary Rutherford and Michael Moneypenny

> In this chapter:
> - Designing the system to encourage patient involvement in their safety and well-being
> - Principles of person-centred care and shared decision making
> - The patient–paramedic interaction
> - Public involvement in service design

Introduction

In safety-critical industries such as aviation, rail and power generation, HF/E principles are aimed at optimising the well-being of the workers in the systems and improving system performance. In addition to the safety and well-being of the worker, enhanced system performance also has positive benefits related to the satisfaction and experience of the consumer or service user. In various ways, members of the public are 'elements of the system' in these industries, for instance, when we fill our cars with fuel, buy transport tickets, operate our home heating systems, or our rare involvement should there be an emergency (using emergency stop buttons on trains and door operation on aircraft). The success of the design of these systems can influence user interaction with these elements.

In healthcare, patients are also 'elements of the system' who interact with other elements, most commonly the healthcare professionals treating or caring for them. Patients are present and often involved in many aspects of their own care, therefore have an opportunity to contribute to their own safety and well-being (Davis et al, 2007). Two of the main ways in which patients and the public could have input into healthcare are:

- interaction with the healthcare workers at the point of care
- involvement in the design of healthcare processes.

This chapter will therefore consider an HF/E approach to the patient's involvement within the pre-hospital system. Why the system should be designed and shaped

Chapter 6 – The Patient: An Element of the System

to encourage patient and service user involvement will be discussed, and how this can contribute to optimising their own safety and well-being. This will lead into discussion regarding how the patient and ambulance clinician interact (primarily in non-life-threatening situations), the benefits of shared decision making, and how you can use a person-centred care approach to facilitate this (note: this is not the same as the person-centred approach to reviewing adverse events). Patient and Public Involvement (PPI) initiatives that engage with patient representatives to facilitate patient and service user input into the design and improvement of healthcare systems will also be considered.

Patient Engagement for Patient Safety

Health and social care systems have traditionally been designed with the patient viewed as a passive participant in the processes, which can inhibit opportunities for patient engagement and contribution to their own safety (Patient Safety Learning, 2019). However, the concept of designing healthcare systems to encourage patients to become more involved in the delivery of care is increasingly evident. This is likely to be in response to reports such as the Berwick review, which asserts that patient safety improves when patients are more involved. The Berwick report states:

> Patient involvement is crucial to the delivery of appropriate, meaningful and safe healthcare and is essential at every stage of the care cycle: at the front line, at the interface between patient and clinician; at the organisational level; at the community level; and at the national level.
>
> (Department of Health, 2013)

Patient involvement is key because, unlike healthcare professionals, patients often see the whole process of their care (Vincent, 2010). This means that the patient has a privileged view that allows them to see the limitations of the healthcare system and notice when things go wrong. This is supported by the World Health Organization (2016) statement that 'when systems open themselves up to patients rather than being reactive, this is likely to improve system efficiency and the quality of care'. Expanding on the two main ways mentioned for patient and public input, Vincent (2010) states that there are several specific times for patient participation in healthcare safety:

- helping to reach an accurate diagnosis
- sharing decisions about treatments and procedures
- contributing to safe medication use
- participating in infection control initiatives
- checking the accuracy of medical records
- observing and checking care processes
- identifying and reporting treatment complications and adverse events

- practising effective self-management (including treatment monitoring)
- shaping the design and improvement of services.

While there are benefits from increasing patient involvement in safety, it is important to appreciate that this will be a significant change from the historical paternalistic approach of healthcare. This may therefore require a shift in culture within some ambulance services. Additionally, engaging patients should only be part of organisational strategies for enhancing patient safety and it is important that it is not perceived as shifting responsibility from the healthcare professional to the patient (Davis et al, 2007).

Person-Centred Care

Person-centred care is 'focusing care on the needs of the individual, ensuring that people's preferences, needs and values guide clinical decisions, and providing care that is respectful of and responsive to them' (Healthcare Education England, 2018). Although the term patient-centred is not new, person-centred care with a focus on shared decision-making is now considered central to healthcare strategies (The Health Foundation, 2016). While the terms 'patient-centred' and 'person-centred' can often be used interchangeably, person-centred is often considered a more contemporary term in relation to health and social care integration, where not all service users are patients. This term also allows us to include patients, carers and relatives in considering their roles within the complex socio-technical system of healthcare.

A person-centred approach puts the person at the heart of healthcare, as is illustrated by the HF/E 'onion' model mentioned in Chapter 1. The SEIPS model discussed in previous chapters also places the patient centrally within the work system, in addition to illustrating how their well-being is an outcome of systems and processes. This demonstrates how and where the patient has a role to play in influencing their own outcomes, and that systems need to be designed to encourage this.

In their Scope of Practice policy, the UK College of Paramedics also supports the adoption of a person-centred approach by stating that paramedics should demonstrate the following competencies regarding the service user relationship:

- performance of a flexible and holistic patient-centred assessment with individualised management plans
- ensure decisions and management plans are in partnership with service users and carers
- facilitation of patients' responsibility and control of their own health and illness
- application of the principles of shared decision making.

(College of Paramedics, 2018)

Chapter 6 – The Patient: An Element of the System

Shared Decision Making

In healthcare, the decision making related to a patient's treatment is often carried out in a paternalistic way, meaning that clinicians can frequently make decisions *for* people rather than *with* them. In pre-hospital care this may involve a traditional approach of the paramedic deciding the best course of action for the patient, based on their assessment of the patient, the options available at that time and their experiences of previous similar situations. This may be understandable if we consider the historical origins of ambulance service provision, where the main aim was to treat patients in life-threatening emergency situations, predominantly requiring this type of decision making. However, in other more routine and non-life-threatening situations, this may create a steep authority gradient which could have negative implications for the involvement of patients in the decision making related to their care. Evidence suggests that patient satisfaction increases when they are involved in the consultation and invited to discuss what matters to them (Shabason et al, 2014).

It is also important to consider the legal implications of not involving patients in decisions related to their care. The Montgomery v Lanarkshire Health Board legal case (2015) is considered a landmark case in relation to informed consent, disclosing the risks of treatment or management decisions to a patient and involving them in such decisions (Box 6.1). Previous tests of informed consent and disclosure had been

---

Box 6.1 – Montgomery v NHS Lanarkshire

Mrs Nadine Montgomery gave birth to a baby boy in October 1999. During delivery, the baby's shoulder became stuck inside her pelvis, a situation known as shoulder dystocia. In the 12 minutes between the baby's head appearing and the baby being fully born, manoeuvres and procedures were being carried out, however the umbilical cord was completely or partially occluded, depriving him of oxygen, which resulted in cerebral palsy.

During her ante-natal care, Mrs Montgomery, who is of small stature and has diabetes, had expressed anxiety and concern to the obstetrician regarding the size of her baby in relation to her ability to give birth. Mrs Montgomery had been told that she was having a large baby, although she was not told about the known increased risks of shoulder dystocia (9–10% of diabetic mothers). The doctor later stated that it was not their normal practice to explain this risk unless specifically asked, as it would likely result in most women requesting a Caesarean section, which they felt was not in women's best interests. Mrs Montgomery successfully argued that if she had known the risk, she would indeed have requested a Caesarean section and her son would not have cerebral palsy.

Ambulance clinicians may not often find themselves being required to explain the risk of shoulder dystocia to pregnant women. However, the landmark Montgomery case is relevant to all healthcare professionals and encourages reflection regarding when and how patients should be and must be involved in decisions related to their own care.

Source: The Supreme Court (2015).

weighted towards the clinicians' professional judgement in disclosing information. However, the Supreme Court judgement in favour of Mrs Montgomery introduced a patient-focused test to UK law.

In shared decision-making, when appropriate, the healthcare professional should seek to outline the options that are available to the patient, explaining the risks and benefits of each. The clinician should make it easy for the patient to explain what is important to them in terms of treatment options and management plan. This approach may not be suitable in all circumstances, therefore will require skilled facilitation and consideration of the factors that can influence it, which are outlined later in this chapter.

The Paramedic–Patient Interaction

As discussed, HF/E is interested in how humans interact with each other. In healthcare application of HF/E, this can tend to focus on interactions between healthcare professions within teams (see Chapter 9). However, ambulance clinicians and patients interact in many situations, from non-time-critical discussion and conversation to life-saving interventions. The Carter report (2018) on performance and unwarranted variations in English NHS Ambulance Trusts states that 'calls for life-threatening emergencies now only make up 10% of demand, with the remainder mostly for patients with urgent primary, social or mental health care needs'. Therefore, in response to this and the earlier point regarding paternalistic decision making in immediately life-threatening emergencies, the focus of this discussion will be on the interactions during calls that are less time-critical. These are also the interactions that will best provide a platform for facilitating shared decision-making approaches.

Patient Consultation

The traditional patient assessment strategy that has been taught in paramedic practice is the widely used catastrophic haemorrhage, airway, breathing, circulation, disability and exposure (<C>ABCDE) structure, which should quickly identify potential life-threatening conditions (JRCALC, 2019). Further assessment, if the situation allows, includes gathering information regarding the patient's illness and 'history' (Box 6.2). This approach to history taking is described as a functional 'medical model' for tackling the problem of what is wrong with the patient, although it is limited in considering wider matters such as the patients' opinion, values, understanding and the effects of their illness on their life (Mehay et al, 2019). This may therefore limit the involvement of the patient in shared decision making.

General Practitioner (GP) teaching and practice involves use of consultation models as an expansion of the traditional medical model. This approach may also be adopted by paramedics when appropriate to enhance the patient's involvement at this stage of interaction. Pawlikowska et al (2002) define a consultation as 'a two-way encounter between a practitioner and a patient', and the use of a model gives a structure to the consultation. There are a few different models, some that are more weighted to what the clinician thinks and decides, and others that are more person-centred. Mehay et al (2019) discuss the benefits and limitations of 14 different

Chapter 6 – The Patient: An Element of the System

> ### Box 6.2 – History-Taking Format
>
> - presenting complaint
> - history of presenting complaint
> - past medical history
> - family history
> - social history
> - drug and allergy history
> - systems review.
>
> *Source:* Joint Royal Colleges Ambulance Liaison Committee, Association of Ambulance Chief Executives (2019).

consultation styles and suggest that Pendleton's model (1984), Neighbour's model (1987) and the Calgary–Cambridge guide (1996, later updated in 2003) have similar weighting of person-centredness. They further state that the Calgary–Cambridge guide (Figure 6.1) is the most favoured model in the UK and is the most evidence-based in relation to communication between clinician and patient. It could therefore be a useful tool to encourage patient participation and engagement at the point of care.

Patients Highlighting When Things Go Wrong

Patients also have a role to play in the detection and prevention of when things go wrong during their care (Unruh and Pratt, 2007). Therefore, in addition to shared decision making, when a professional relationship and rapport is achieved, the patient could potentially be involved in other aspects of their care related to adverse events if enabled to do so. It is important to acknowledge that there may be a reluctance from the patient to raise concerns or ask a question, and that both patients and healthcare professionals may consider this as challenging the clinicians' professionalism. Pre-hospital examples could include handovers and checking of patient care records.

Handovers

Good handover of information between clinicians is associated with improved patient safety (Wood et al, 2014). The paramedic-to-receiving clinician handover can often take place in busy, distracting and non-confidential environments, and may also occur without the presence of the patient or their family. Any of these factors could create a situation where important information is not passed on, and the patient is unable to correct the omission or mistake. Taking time to design the work system interactions related to handovers, including an appropriate environment, a shallow authority gradient with the patient, and inviting the patient to listen to the handover, could result in enhanced safety during this process.

Factors That Influence Patient Participation

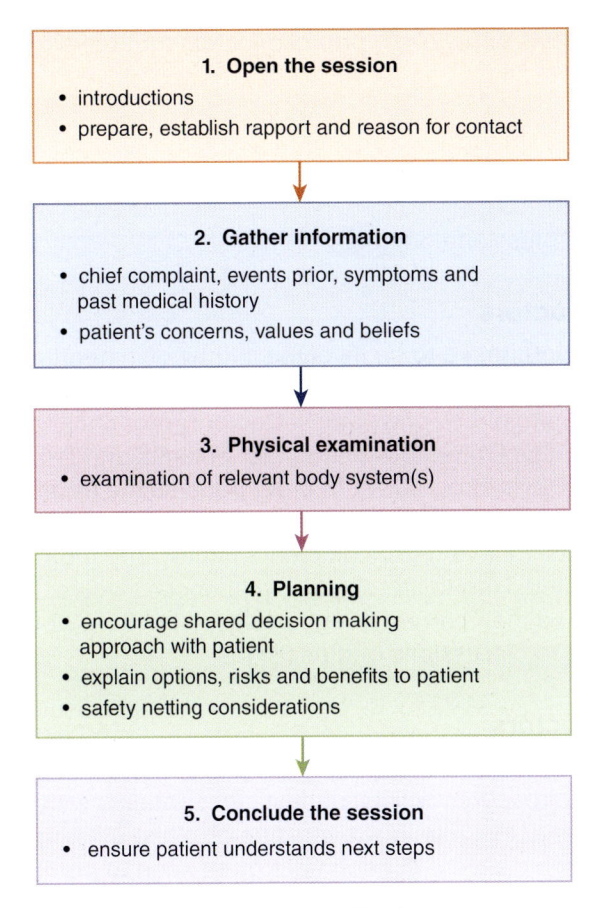

1. Open the session
- introductions
- prepare, establish rapport and reason for contact

2. Gather information
- chief complaint, events prior, symptoms and past medical history
- patient's concerns, values and beliefs

3. Physical examination
- examination of relevant body system(s)

4. Planning
- encourage shared decision making approach with patient
- explain options, risks and benefits to patient
- safety netting considerations

5. Conclude the session
- ensure patient understands next steps

Figure 6.1 – Principles of Calgary–Cambridge Guide
Source: Based on Silverman et al (2013)

Checking Patient Care Records

Patients are entitled to review any documentation related to their care and doing so may also provide opportunity for the patient to spot any errors or inaccuracies that have been documented. Ambulance clinicians could therefore invite patients to review care records for accuracy and completeness. This is especially useful when patients are being discharged from scene with self-care advice. The shared review of the patient care record can also serve as a recap and to check the patient's understanding of care provided, safety netting advice and other elements relating to the non-conveyance.

Factors That Influence Patient Participation

Although patient participation in their own safety is desirable, there are factors and influences that must be considered, as not all patients will be willing or able to contribute. Davis et al (2007) propose factors that are likely to influence participation:

- patient-related factors
- illness-related factors
- healthcare professional factors.

Patient-Related Factors

The patient's ability and desire to be involved in their own healthcare may be variable depending on circumstances, for example, cognitive ability, stress, severity of illness, previous experiences and values. Demographic characteristics can also influence the level of involvement, with younger patients and females opting for more input into their care (Davis et al, 2007). In older patients the traditional view of 'the clinician knows best' may still often be the case. Therefore, an invitation extended to a patient to express their views or comment on their care may not always be accepted as anticipated. Health literacy also influences involvement, as the more a patient can understand their current health position, the more able and willing they may be to contribute to discussions and decisions.

Illness-Related Factors

The severity and presentation of illness or injury needs to be considered. Davis et al (2007) highlight some research which suggests that patients with minor illness are more likely to play an active role, however, they also cite evidence which suggests that patients with chronic severe ill health are often keen to participate in their care and that this can benefit the long-term management of their illness.

In terms of medical emergencies, Vincent (2010) suggests that acutely unwell patients often leave all immediate decisions to healthcare staff. This may be because patients who present as emergencies have limited understanding regarding what is wrong with them and find it harder to engage in their care. However, Vincent and Coulter (2002) state that it may be important to ascertain the views and wishes of patients even during critical illness to ensure those wishes are considered.

Prior experience can also play a part in a patient's desire to contribute. If someone has a new experience of ill health, for example, their first episode of chest pain, they may find it more difficult to engage than someone who has experienced a number of episodes of chest pain and has an understanding of their condition.

Paramedic Factors

The knowledge, skills and attitudes of ambulance clinicians are important factors in influencing patient engagement. Recognising the benefit of patient involvement, knowing when it should be encouraged and how to facilitate it are essential to its success. Patients will understandably have concerns and may find it difficult to challenge a healthcare professional or to speak up about their concerns if it is not made easy for them to do so. Patients need to feel comfortable that their wishes and concerns will be listened to and not dismissed. One of the main factors required to facilitate shared decision making is a trusting relationship. If this can be established, then both the paramedic and the patient (or their family) will feel comfortable and able to freely discuss their views to achieve an agreed goal.

Public Involvement in Co-Design and Service Improvement

Patients, service users, their families and lay people should also be involved in improving the quality of healthcare through partnership arrangements with healthcare providers (NHS England, 2019). Carman et al (2013) state that patient engagement is an essential part of a healthcare provider's continuous learning, and essential for the re-design of healthcare services. People can improve system performance by taking part in Patient and Public Involvement (PPI) or Patient Safety Partner (PSP) initiatives which facilitate public input in decisions related to healthcare design, service delivery and improvements. Potential roles for public involvement are:

- training, education and recruitment of healthcare staff
- service and pathway design
- review of complaints
- participation in patient safety investigations
- members of safety, quality and audit committees
- learning from patient experience
- policy development.

(NHS England, 2019)

Active involvement in co-design and service improvement will require concerted effort and commitment on the part of the ambulance service to reach out and engage with patients and their families. This can often be challenging due to the short periods of time that patients can spend in the care of pre-hospital providers and the challenges of making contact after care provision. Ambulance services often have patient and public representation in aspects of their governance processes, although more work needs done to further implement involvement in healthcare (NHS England, 2019; Patient Safety Learning, 2019). NHS England (2017) recommend:

- encouraging and respecting different beliefs and opinions
- specifically seeking input from those who experience health inequalities and poor health outcomes
- valuing people's lived experiences
- providing clear and easy-to-understand information
- working with advocacy services where required

Chapter 6 – The Patient: An Element of the System

- being open, honest and transparent
- avoiding tokenism
- reviewing positive and negative experiences and learning from them.

Always Events

The 'always event' concept is an innovative approach to engage with patients to improve their healthcare experiences through re-design of the system. Always events are agreed aspects of a patient's care experience that are deemed so important to them that they must always occur on a consistent basis for every patient (Picker Institute, 2020).

The process of implementing an always event involves selecting a specific patient group, then engaging with the group to understand what is important to them, possibly through interviews or questionnaires. Processes are then put in place to measure how often the always event occurs. A key principle to always events is that the patient and their families are involved in the identification and co-production of the event that matters to them. The productive partnerships between patients and healthcare providers enable the co-design of solutions to improve patient experience and outcome.

Simple examples of always events may be:

- healthcare staff always introduce themselves
- patients always know what is going to happen next
- patients are always treated with dignity and respect.

Always events could possibly be considered the opposite of 'never events' that are established in some healthcare systems (Bowie et al, 2015). Never events are discussed in Chapter 10.

Feedback Systems

Gaining feedback from the patient on the delivery of healthcare also provides information to allow improvements to be made. Feedback mechanisms can often be questionnaires or surveys, although social media and online platforms are increasingly recognised as ways of engaging with the public and gathering feedback on service delivery experiences. Care Opinion is a community interest company recognised by the NHS in Scotland and England. It provides an online platform that allows service users and their families to provide feedback on their care. The organisations then engage with the patient by providing a response online and sharing how learning has taken place to strengthen the work system. One must bear in mind, however, that over-reliance on a web-based feedback system may lead to large segments of the population being overlooked, such as those with limited internet connectivity or digital literacy.

Summary

Key principles in the application of HF/E approaches are understanding the interactions between elements of the system and design of the system in response to that understanding. The patient and the ambulance clinician are key elements in a pre-hospital work system, with communication and shared decision making between them influencing patient experiences and outcomes. Harnessing the added value of input from the patient within the system may require changes in individual practice and at organisational levels for ambulance services. Systems can be shaped, strengthened and designed to encourage patient involvement, and the benefits of including the patient are manifold with the return on investment contributing to increased patient satisfaction and safety.

References

Bowie, P. et al. (2015). Quality improvement and person-centredness: a participatory mixed methods study to develop the 'always event' concept for primary care. *British Medical Journal Open*. 5: 1–8.

Care Opinion (2020). Care opinion: what's your story? [online]. Available from: https://www.careopinion.org.uk/

Carman, K.L. et al. (2013). Patient and family engagement: a framework for understanding the elements and developing interventions and policies. *Health Affairs (Project Hope)*. 32(2): 223–231.

Carter, P. (2018). Operational productivity and performance in English NHS Ambulance Trusts: unwarranted variations [online]. Available from: https://improvement.nhs.uk/documents/3271/Operational_productivity_and_performance_NHS_Ambulance_Trusts_final.pdf

College of Paramedics (2018). Paramedic – Scope of Practice Policy [online]. Bridgwater: College of Paramedics. Available from: https://collegeofparamedics.co.uk/COP/Professional Development/Scope_of_Practice.aspx

Davis, R.E. et al. (2007). Patient involvement in patient safety: what factors influence patient participation and engagement? *Health Expectations* [online]. 10: 259–267. Available from: https://www.ncbi.nlm.nih.gov/pubmed/17678514

Department of Health (2013). A promise to learn – a commitment to act [online]. London: Williams Lea. Available from: https://assets.publishing.service.gov.uk/government/uploads/system/uploads/attachment_data/file/226703/Berwick_Report.pdf

Healthcare Education England (2018). Person-centred care [online]. Available from: https://www.hee.nhs.uk/our-work/person-centred-care

Joint Royal Colleges Ambulance Liaison Committee, Association of Ambulance Chief Executives (2019). *JRCALC Clinical Guidelines 2019*. Bridgwater: Class Professional Publishing.

Mehay, R. et al. (2019). Revisiting models of the consultation [online]. Available from: https://www.essentialgptrainingbook.com/wp-content/online-resources/04%20consultation%20models.pdf

Montgomery v Lanarkshire Health Board (2015). https://www.supremecourt.uk/cases/docs/uksc-2013-0136-judgment.pdf

NHS England (2017). Patient and public participation policy [online]. Available from: https://www.england.nhs.uk/wp-content/uploads/2017/04/ppp-policy.pdf

Chapter 6 – The Patient: An Element of the System

NHS England (2019). The NHS patient safety strategy: safer culture, safer systems, safer patients [online]. Available from: https://improvement.nhs.uk/documents/5472/190708_Patient_Safety_Strategy_for_website_v4.pdf

Patient Safety Learning (2019). The patient-safe future: a blueprint for action [online]. Available from: https://s3-eu-west-1.amazonaws.com/ddme-psl/content/A-Blueprint-for-Action-240619.pdf?mtime=20190701143409&focal=none

Pawlikowska, T. et al. (2002). Consultation models. In: Charlton, R. (ed.). *Learning to Consult*. Boca Raton: CRC Press, pp. 178–215.

Picker Institute (2020). Always events® [online]. Available from: https://www.picker.org/always-events/

Shabason, J.E. et al. (2014). Shared decision-making and patient control in radiation oncology: implications for patient satisfaction. *Cancer*. 120(12): 1863–1870.

Silverman, J. et al. (2013). Skills for Communicating with Patients. 3rd Ed. Boca Raton: CRC Press.

The Health Foundation (2016). Person-centred care made simple [online]. London: The Health Foundation. Available from: https://www.health.org.uk/sites/default/files/PersonCentredCareMadeSimple.pdf

Unruh, K.T., Pratt, W. (2007). Patients as actors: the patient's role in detecting, preventing, and recovering from medical errors. *International Journal of Medical Informatics*. 76(Suppl 1): S236–S244.

Vincent, C. (2010). *Patient Safety*. 2nd Ed. West Sussex: Wiley-Blackwell.

Vincent, C.A., Coulter, A. (2002). Patient safety: what about the patient? *Quality & Safety in Health Care*. 11(1): 76–80.

Wood, K. et al. (2014). Clinical handovers between prehospital and hospital staff: literature review. *Emergency Medical Journal*. 32: 577–581.

World Health Organization (2016). Patient engagement [online]. Available from: https://apps.who.int/iris/bitstream/handle/10665/252269/9789241511629-eng.pdf;jsessionid=C34C43BD07FE208CBFA2046507136AC6?sequence=1

Chapter 7
Well-Being of the Paramedic

Jo Mildenhall

In this chapter:
- Workplace well-being in the context of HF/E
- Relationship between well-being and system performance
- Brief theory of stress and influencing factors related to emergency responders
- A systems-thinking approach to mediating and managing stress and well-being

Introduction

Enhancing well-being is one of the main aims of adopting an HF/E approach when understanding and designing a system, the other aim being optimising system performance. By using a systems-thinking approach to better understand the relationship and close influences between system performance and well-being, ambulance services can cultivate a healthy, productive workplace while simultaneously delivering quality patient care that is safe and effective.

Mental well-being and occupational stress are currently very topical across various industries due in part to the general rise in numbers of employees experiencing mental ill health in the workplace. As a result, it seems that greater emphasis is being placed upon maintaining the wellness of employed people than ever before.

Rather than seeking to understand mental ill-health as a collection of signs and symptoms which affect individuals, and which they are encouraged to personally manage, an HF/E perspective considers how the design of a workplace and the interactions between elements within it influence employees' well-being, either as individuals or as a collective. Within the professional healthcare setting of paramedicine, this HF/E focused approach to well-being appears to have had limited consideration in previously published research. In order to fill this gap, this chapter provides an understanding of how occupational work systems, particularly those associated with the pre-hospital environment, influence well-being. Furthermore, the chapter also details how developing a knowledge of the interactions between individuals and elements of the work system can actually enable us to broaden our understanding of the impact upon well-being.

Well-Being in the Workplace

The World Health Organization's definition of health as 'a state of complete physical, mental and social well-being, and not merely the absence of disease or infirmity' (2013) firmly recognises the importance of well-being in the context of good health. However, arguably well-being is much more, encompassing a sense of positivity, satisfaction and purpose in life, and feeling socially connected (Department of Health, 2013). Well-being may be viewed as a holistic concept, considering the individual as a whole for whom there is influence and interaction from a wide variety of factors – including that of employment. Psychosocial dynamics are also important elements of the workplace which can contribute to employee well-being. These include team working, social/peer support, leadership styles and job fulfilment, whereby employees influence the working environment, as well as the occupational culture and the way the work gets done. The psychosocial benefits of work are noted, with Waddell and Burton (2006) specifically highlighting the positive influence upon an individual's sense of self, personal and professional identity, as well as their economic and social status. They particularly emphasise the importance of work in providing an opportunity to meet psychosocial needs by reducing feelings of isolation and bringing pleasure from shared social networking and communications. While these benefits of working may seem obvious, Javaid et al (2017) commented that a negative psychosocial work environment can also be detrimental to employee health and wellness. Such a work environment could be one where a person feels alone in the workplace, perceives excessive pressures and demands, finds their work unmanageable or difficult, or perhaps not challenging and stimulating enough. These work environments have been associated with depression, anxiety, stress, burnout and reduced self-esteem within staff. Furthermore, Black (2012) stated that 'there is strong evidence that prolonged loss of work, whatever the cause, can harm physical and mental health' which may lead to 'increased risk of mortality and morbidity ... cardiovascular disease, poor mental health, suicide and health-damaging behaviours' (Public Health England, 2019a). Therefore, it follows that being in work is regarded as better for an individual's well-being than being unemployed.

Importantly, recent guidance from Public Health England (2019b) clarified that for work to promote well-being, it must be perceived positively by the individual, with key determinants being employment safety and security, good working conditions such as hours and pay, opportunities for development and learning, and a supportive environment with access to appropriate welfare and health facilities such as occupational health and physiotherapy.

Employee health and well-being is fundamental in contributing to – and influencing – an individual's behaviours, emotional responses and cognitive processes. This includes situation awareness and decision making, with risk markedly increased where those decisions involve the weighing up and consideration of complex factors, and which have the potential to impact upon system performance and subsequent patient/public safety (Reid and Bromiley, 2012).

Well-Being, Work Processes and System Performance

As discussed, the HF/E approach allows us to understand those interactive elements within a workplace environment which influence system performance and well-being (Bennett et al, 2005; Carayon et al, 2014a). This perspective not only enables us to seek effective solutions to improve employee health and well-being, but also to deliver safe, high-quality care.

Employees are absolutely key to the reliability and performance of systems within the workplace (Reason, 2008), and in the health arena such systems include patient care and management. HF/E recognises the importance of workers, although, as discussed in Chapters 2 and 5, advocates the perspective that work systems and processes should be designed to adapt to individuals rather than the other way around. Dul et al (2012) stated that when a systems approach is adopted to design the work elements, the well-being of the employees can be optimised in terms of:

- enhanced physical, psychological and social well-being
- increased motivation, growth, learning and job satisfaction
- improved performance.

A poorly designed system of work can result in negative stress and/or mental ill-health (WHO, 2009) leading to increased sickness absence and/or reduced ability to function. Alternatively, employees may feel pressured to continue to attend work despite feeling unwell (presenteeism) (Black, 2012; Stevenson and Farmer, 2017). These staff members are also likely to experience chronic stress and associated mental ill health, as well as physical ill health including chronic musculoskeletal injuries and/or cardiovascular disease. Clearly this is detrimental to the individual, but also has a wider impact upon family, colleagues, service users, patients, the organisation for whom they work and the broader social economy.

Within the ambulance service sector, workplace systems that may influence well-being and system performance include technical procedures, working hours and shift patterns, supervision and feedback mechanisms, operational demand, education and professional development, teamwork and the work environment. Possessing an awareness of HF/E in terms of behaviours, an individual's physical and psychological limitations, and understanding the characteristics of systems, could help to identify the need to improve and strengthen workplace systems. A re-design may include examining how tasks and procedures are implemented and how work is organised (such as shift patterns, relief working, flexibility to alter working hours).

Crucially, it is in the interest of organisations to optimise employee well-being to facilitate a more productive, engaged and motivated workforce who will likely have greater attendance at work, leading to improved system performance.

Well-Being in the Pre-Hospital System

The demand upon emergency ambulance services has continued to increase year-upon-year (NHS England, 2018a) placing growing pressure upon those who work

Chapter 7 – Well-Being of the Paramedic

within the pre-hospital system. Both within the UK and internationally (such as in Australia and New Zealand), system performance and effective service delivery has been explicitly measured in terms of emergency response times. More recently, however, there has been additional focus on clinical effectiveness and clinical outcomes via audit and research study (NHS England, 2018b), but within occupational and academic spheres, it is only within the last few years that we have seen increased attention on the health and well-being of ambulance staff. Nevertheless, it is imperative that both organisations and professional bodies – particularly in safety-critical industries such as the emergency services – invest in the well-being of their people. For ambulance services, this is particularly relevant given the professional responsibility of paramedics in providing safe clinical care.

Indeed, pre-hospital care systems offer a somewhat unique working environment and one that is challenging to design in such a way that all elements interact to optimise staff well-being. As previously noted, the system is almost always under high demand, with the frequent occurrence of unpredictable variation and risk. It is an occupation in which the work is often intense, including:

- decision making relating to a multitude of clinical presentations, often involving patients with complex social, psychological and medical needs
- a pace of work which can be variable but in which the service is frequently under significant demand
- long working hours and shift work often with enforced overtime (late finishes), which subsequently impacts upon time for rest and recuperation
- exposure to the 'emotional intensity' of distressing, traumatic and sometimes high-risk situations (McFarlane and Bryant, 2007; Maguire et al, 2014; Granter et al, 2019)
- undertaking high-level concentration skills such as emergency driving, often over long distances (Corman, 2017).

Thus, there is a requirement that staff working within this field are sufficiently both physically and psychologically well to undertake the role. The mental well-being of emergency services employees, however, is of particular concern. Psychological ill health is reported as the leading cause of sickness absence among frontline NHS ambulance staff, with current figures being far greater than that of other occupational healthcare groups or indeed, that of the general population. Through survey results, the mental health charity MIND (2019) noted that of 'blue light' respondents, 88% of emergency services personnel had experienced poor mental health and stress while employed within this field. More specifically, a systematic review and meta-analysis conducted by Petrie et al (2018a) of prevalence rates of post-traumatic stress disorder (PTSD) and mental health conditions among ambulance personnel identified that, of 30,878 staff, the average prevalence rate for PTSD was 11% (in comparison to 3% of the general population). Depression was reported by 15% of those surveyed, and anxiety a further 15%. However, it is arguable that, as a result of continued stigma around mental health conditions both within society and ambulance/emergency services organisational culture, there may be additional staff who are reluctant to disclose distress and psychological fatigue and ill health for fear of occupational demise and negative impact upon their professional self-image and careers. Thus, the numbers of ambulance staff suffering across the globe may be considerably higher.

Of particular concern is the rise in suicides among this population. Hird et al (2019) reviewed details pertaining to completed suicides among paramedics in England between 2011 and 2015. The researchers found that male paramedics were 75% more at risk of suicide than the general population, with males in their early forties most at risk. It was not understood from the study why the paramedics had ended their life, therefore we cannot be clear that work was a significant, contributing factor. In collaboration with the Association of Ambulance Chief Executives (AACE), recommendations from this study include educating all employees on how to recognise and respond to a co-worker who may be distressed, and a call to review occupational health and counselling facilities available in all English Ambulance NHS Trusts (AACE, 2018a).

At a national level within the UK, NHS Horizons partnering with AACE has taken a systems approach to explore positive improvements to system re-design in NHS Ambulance Services. Known as 'Project A', this innovative programme sought to understand from frontline staff their ideas on what can make a difference to urgent and emergency healthcare services. Over 500 ideas were generated and these were encapsulated within 16 themes, one of which was improving the well-being and mental health of ambulance staff (AACE, 2018b). Through social media, ambulance staff from across the nation highlighted that focus was needed to:

- promote staff well-being and access to well-being support
- open conversations around mental health
- facilitate debriefs (defusing) after significant incidents
- create time and space for rest and relaxation
- support continuing professional development
- create clear career and development opportunities for all.

In summary of Project A, it may be proposed that an HF/E, systems thinking approach could be adopted to improve the design of the pre-hospital work system to incorporate these ideas to enhance staff well-being. While improving the interactive elements of the work system is a way to optimise whole system performance and human well-being, such improvements can only occur with awareness of when well-being is adversely affecting individuals and groups working within an organisation.

Occupational Stress

Stress may be defined as an individual's response of psychological strain or tension to a threat, or excessive demands or pressures which are perceived by the individual as outweighing their own personal resources or capabilities at that time (MIND, 2013; Health and Safety Executive, 2019).

Chapter 7 – Well-Being of the Paramedic

In the context of workplace well-being, stress has been identified as significantly influential upon an individual's physical and mental health. Indeed, stress is a leading cause of poor mental health and well-being of ambulance staff. NHS Digital (2019) reported that between July 2017 and June 2018, 20.8% of sickness in all Ambulance Trusts in England were attributed to stress. This equates to one in five working days, with 50,031 full-time equivalent days lost. There was 1.09% overall difference between the highest and lowest reported rates of stress-related sickness absence.

Understanding work-related stress, however, requires a holistic approach which reflects the complexity of individual differences and takes account of human interactions, experience and occupational exposure.

Considerable depth of research has been undertaken into the negative influences and outcomes of experiences of stressful stimuli; particularly around the physiological impact upon health and well-being. This may, in part, reflect a western world view based upon the medical model of disease and dysfunction, which has subsequently framed our understanding of the concept of stress in terms of symptoms, cause and effect (Yaribeygi et al, 2017). However, this is not the only perspective.

Contemporary psychology has drawn upon Selye's (1974) work on 'eustress' to understand stress as a positive adaption of human functioning and performance within the workplace. Essentially, eustress may be regarded as an 'adaptive', healthy, positive response to perceived stressful stimuli (Lazarus, 1993) which is associated with improved performance, positive affective state (emotional response), feelings of meaningfulness, positive engagement and satisfaction, and having a sense of hope (McGowan et al, 2006). For paramedics, this may also include feelings of 'a job well done', contentment at being able to utilise one's clinical skills, and contributing to improving patient outcomes. Distress, on the other hand, (a non-adaptive form of stress where negative emotions are felt) has been linked with feelings such as anger and frustration, increased anxiety and physical reactions such as poor sleep, reduced appetite and use of maladaptive coping strategies such as increased alcohol intake. It would appear that organisational literature to date contains little discussion on the concepts and interrelationships between stress, distress and eustress (Kupriyanov and Zhdanov, 2014).

In contrast, psychosocial perspectives validate the influence of psychosocial, cultural and emotional processes in an individual's interpretation, experience and response to stressful situations. Within this context, stress may be viewed as a challenge to our emotional and psychological safety, disrupting our perceptions, thoughts and beliefs about people or situations in our lives which we take to be our normal reality.

Central to the way in which an individual experiences a stressful stimulus is the perception they have of that stressor within the context of other factors such as perceived control/lack of control, persistence of the stress, and whether the stressor is desired. These variables (and others) will likely determine how the individual interprets the stressful situation and responds to it. Such a process is highly complex and multifactorial, which may leave the individual experiencing a range of emotions and responses concurrently. For example, in paramedic practice, attending to a critically unwell patient involved in a significant road traffic collision may bring about the perception and interpretation of the incident as being a stressor due to the intensity and timeliness of clinical care required. Subsequently, the paramedic may feel initially overwhelmed at being confronted by the multiple tasks that need to be undertaken rapidly, yet they may also experience eustress at being able to use their knowledge and clinical skills to provide effective patient care.

In terms of HF/E, it is important to highlight that adverse exposure to stress (whether acute or chronic) has been linked with reduced system performance through, for example, work absence and the inability of individuals (and teams) to complete tasks which would previously have been within their capability.

Maslow's Hierarchy of Needs

Very relevant to our understanding of stress within the workplace is Maslow's (1943, 1962) Hierarchy of Needs theory (Figure 7.1) which explains that for psychological motivation and fulfilment, basic needs must be adequately met before an individual can attend to more complex situations. While there are various critiques of this model which are beyond the scope of this chapter, fundamentally, this theory suggests that physiological and safety needs, such as having time and access to somewhere safe and secure to rest, and having access to nourishing food and warmth, are imperative before psychological and self-fulfilment (personal growth) needs can be attended to. Challenges to these needs are likely to result in stress, leading to decreased motivation, an increased feeling of pressure and reduced engagement of employees.

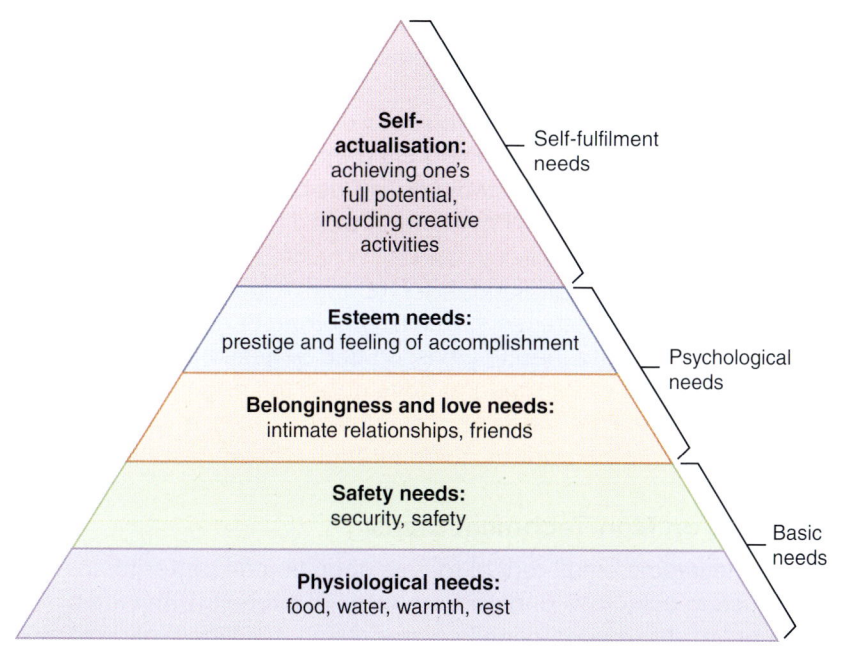

Figure 7.1 – Maslow's Hierarchy of Needs
Source: Based on image from Factoryjoe via Wikimedia Commons: https://commons.wikimedia.org/wiki/File:Mazlow%27s_Hierarchy_of_Needs.svg

Chapter 7 – Well-Being of the Paramedic

Although dependent on personal circumstances and individual differences, Maslow proposed that the following are key needs which must be more-or-less met before more complex needs may be attended to:

- **Physiological** – having access to water, food, shelter, and being able to have adequate rest and sleep.
- **Safety and security** – having stable employment which provides psychological fulfilment, a safe and secure environment to live and work in, financial security, meeting the needs of any personal health issues.
- **Belongingness** – having a sense of connection with others, family, friends and colleagues, not feeling isolated, or having a negative experience of being alone.
- **Esteem** – possessing self-esteem, recognition and status from life/work, having the freedom to make choices without coercion.
- **Self-actualisation** – having the freedom, autonomy, empowerment and desire to be the best that one can be, to work towards and achieve goals and ambitions.

Sources of Stress

The sources of stress and the personal impact can significantly differ between individuals depending on a host of variables including, but not limited to, previous experiences, personal relationship circumstances, the social environment, general physical and psychological health at the time of the stress, access to social support and even our genetic make-up. Specifically, for emergency services personnel, work system elements associated with inducing stress are highlighted in Box 7.1.

These factors have the potential to cause stress either in the short term (such as in the case of a situation activating an immediate fear response of fight/flight/freeze) or long term (chronic) in response to multiple demands being placed upon a person or multiple stresses being experienced over a protracted length of time.

As discussed, studies have determined that ambulance staff experience a variety of specific occupational related stressors, which singularly or collectively may increase the risk of deteriorating mental health (Jonsson and Segesten, 2003; Bounds, 2006). Most recently, the College of Paramedics have noted the negative psychological impact of fitness-to-practice hearings on members and have set up dedicated peer-support provision to assist colleagues going through this process (Hancox, 2019).

Impact of Stress on Non-Technical Skills

Understanding the impact of influential factors upon human performance is imperative to system outcomes and performance. Of interest within the pre-hospital field is the impact of stress upon cognitive processing abilities relating to situation awareness, decision making, safe practices for patient care and staff safety, communication and team working (Carayon et al, 2014b). Indeed, the effect of stress upon a paramedic's judgement and cognitive capability is an understated aspect

Box 7.1 – Work System Elements Associated with Stress in Emergency Medical Services Work

- Clinical challenges (Bounds, 2006)
- Being responsible for someone's life
- Providing quality care and performance in the face of time pressures (Jurisova, 2016)
- Legal/professional accountability
- Environmental conditions – weather, violence, fire, darkness
- Lack of/inadequate/defective technology, equipment and resources (Aasa et al, 2005; Jenner, 2007; Jurisova, 2016)
- Moral pressure to take action (Murray et al, 2018)
- Distressing and emotionally intense scenes (Regehr et al, 2002)
- Uncertainty about the situation to be faced – if information is limited about the nature of the incident to be attended this will lead to low levels of situation awareness and uncertainty about potential risks to safety (National Operational Guidance, 2017a)
- Feeling vulnerable – difficult situation to manage at scene, limited/no back-up, fear of danger/injury/assault
- High intensity and demanding workload (National Operational Guidance, 2017a)
- Fatigue – long hours, long run of shifts, night working, working while unwell (presenteeism)
- Performance anxiety – feeling fearful when required to attend an incident which we don't feel clinically confident in dealing with or undertaking a role within which we have little/no experience (National Operational Guidance, 2017a)
- New or unusual situations – where we have 'no experience or recognised procedures to draw on to decide what actions are appropriate' (National Operational Guidance, 2017a)
- Our expectations are not met – 'an incident that alters in an unexpected way, or where indicators of progress or incident type do not fit with current situation awareness. Also, system, procedural, or equipment failures, or human error may result in a plan not being implemented in accordance with expectations' (National Operational Guidance, 2017a)
- Multiple goals – 'complex incidents may generate critical situations that require more than one goal to be addressed, resulting in conflicts between objectives including those of other agencies. This may lead to indecision and hesitation about prioritisation and the actions to be taken' (National Operational Guidance, 2017a)
- Organisational relationships – such as limited leadership/manager/peer support (Sterud et al, 2011)
- Work/life imbalance.

to consider, particularly given the potential impact upon others' lives. However, by understanding how stress affects pre-hospital clinicians, and designing work processes with this in mind, undesired outcomes can be minimised.

While as previously noted, experiencing some stress can help motivate us and enhance our cognitive abilities, at other times, stress can become harmful and may negatively impact us. Poor concentration and decreased alertness may result from the overwhelming pressure associated with stress, thus affecting an individual's perception of the situation and capacity to process working memories. Therefore, stress may inhibit our ability to appraise all information available to us which can inadvertently lead to risk taking and suboptimal decision making. In drawing upon the discussions in Chapters 8 and 9 on situation awareness, decision making and teamwork, it is recognised that stress may impact upon the paramedic in the following ways:

- Impaired situation awareness – 'impairments such as a narrow focus and becoming easily distracted may result in difficulties with scanning the scene. [Paramedics] may struggle to assimilate [new] information presented so that they can understand the situation fully'.

- Impaired decision making – paramedics may fail to 'consider all the relevant issues' due to experiencing 'tunnel vision' which can lead to 'poor decisions being made'. Stress hormones can not only impact upon the perception and interpretation of information, but can also affect behavioural reaction times. Hypervigilance may also affect decision making.

- Impaired communication – poor communication will likely affect team working, leading to a lack of shared understanding about the incident, objectives and plan. Stress may result in auditory exclusion and information overload therefore affecting the ability to process information.

- Impaired performance – affecting both individuals and the team with increased risk of mistakes being made with potential impact on patient safety.

- Impaired leadership – 'negative emotional responses are likely to be detected by others and are known to elicit similar emotions'. This can affect the relationship between colleagues and confidence in abilities may be lost.

(National Operational Guidance Programme, 2017b)

Systems Approaches to Managing Stress and Well-Being

The benefits and challenges of adopting a systems-thinking approach were discussed in Chapter 4. Those principles align to the discussion in this chapter by encouraging consideration of work system interactions upon well-being rather than focusing on individuals only.

In taking a systems interaction approach to mediating and managing stress, the Stevenson and Farmer (2017) 'Thriving at work' independent review of mental health and employers made recommendations for developing knowledge of workplace system factors which influence mental well-being. Supported by Health Education England (2019), one such factor specifically noted was the need to develop awareness of psychological health within the workplace through both education and training for workers and managers, and also through monitoring systems. It is important that such education includes the distinction between normal and problematic responses to stress, and psychological illnesses such as post-traumatic stress disorder (PTSD) (Williams et al, 2014). If an awareness of psychological health can be incorporated into system design, the benefits should subsequently be realised in the outcomes of system performance and well-being.

Designing the system to allow sharing of experiences, knowledge, understanding and best practice around stress and mental health conditions is paramount to enhancing a supportive, inclusive and accepting occupational culture, free from stigma and judgement. However, to do so requires psychological safety and trust – for the employee and employer – particularly around accepting human capabilities and limitations, and it is this that can take time to build within the psycho-relational context of an occupational culture. On this note, Jenner (2007) emphasised that 'formally recognising the potential stress reactions that emergency responders may experience in this way helps to validate and normalise them and this can decrease the emotional fallout of participating in an emergency response as these reactions are no longer hidden, minimised or ridiculed'. Furthermore, possessing awareness and genuine understanding of the impact of stress not only encourages but empowers individuals to disclose when their ability to complete their role is impaired through mental ill health (should they be aware of it), and may increase their confidence to have conversations with other people when they do not feel that they are their usual selves.

Importantly, if stress is not recognised or acknowledged, it could lead to underestimating any potential risks within the systems and processes of work, leading to affected system performance, patient safety risk and poor service experience. Currently the International Paramedic Anxiety Wellbeing and Stress (IPAWS) study is in progress and may help to provide more detailed understanding around the complexities of stress and distress in pre-hospital care (Asbury et al, 2018).

While realistically employers are unable to remove every workplace stressor, particularly within the emergency services for the reasons discussed, managers and leaders are central in optimising employee well-being and system performance by influencing a shift in organisational culture around stress and promoting well-being outcomes (Public Health England, 2019a). They are key to humanising the workplace by taking account of the way workplaces are designed around employees, so that an organisation competently and transparently reduces stress, and supports and helps its employees to cope in an authentic and meaningful way, rather than a superficial tick-box approach (Smith, 2018). This is supported by Petrie et al's (2018b) study drawing upon the experiences of 1622 ambulance employees across two states of Australia, which found that manager support was a 'significant predictor' and a 'potentially modifiable factor influencing employee mental health'. They identified that in addition to managerial behaviours, it was the organisational culture which had a 'substantial influence' on ambulance employee mental well-being. The authors suggested that working conditions, routines, policies and procedures are usually instigated and/or influenced by managers and subsequently inform cultural behaviours and practices (of both employees and managers), which impact upon working conditions and, thus, psychological health. They concluded that commitment to employee psychological well-being is required from senior leaders within the organisation, and consideration needs to be applied to developing 'manager-based approaches' which enhance their ability to provide meaningful and appropriate support to staff.

Undoubtedly, developing an organisational strategy with senior leadership and board-level buy-in, that recognises the influences of workplace factors in the design and process of work systems, is critical to enhancing occupational well-being and reducing stress and distress. However, such a framework needs to be sufficiently flexible to be able to take into account the individual differences of employees and the various influencing factors upon cognitive functioning and coping. While embedding and sustaining well-being improvement initiatives may incur challenges to public sector organisational capabilities and demands, the balance of re-designing workplaces in this way will improve and optimise the health and well-being of individuals and organisations (NHS England, 2018c) and bring enhanced system performance.

Fatigue

Like stress, fatigue has been identified as an influencer upon the well-being of paramedics. Indeed, Paterson et al (2014) highlighted that fatigue was found to be a contributory factor in depression, stress, anxiety, burnout, headaches, gastro-intestinal upset and subsequent absence from work.

An agreed academic definition of fatigue can be difficult to source, although it is generally accepted to be related to a state of tiredness or sleepiness, with three direct causes:

1. extended periods of being awake and reduced sleep
2. wake and sleep patterns that are out of synchrony with our circadian rhythms
3. task factors related to workload and long hours of work.

The fatigue of pre-hospital care providers has also been identified as influencing an individual's cognitive function, affecting situation awareness, decision making,

Circadian rhythm – the 'internal body clock' that regulates the approximately 24-hour cycle of biological processes (Flin et al, 2008).

performance of technical and motor skills, and communication (Flin et al, 2008). Detrimental functioning in these areas has the potential to affect personal safety and add risks to the care given to patients. In their study of operational paramedics, Patterson et al (2012) noted that an increase in personal injury, reporting of adverse events and safety-compromising behaviours was found among fatigued paramedics, compared with those who were non-fatigued.

Paterson et al (2014) researched paramedic views on causes of fatigue that are specific to them, and describe a number of 'indirect contributors', most of which you are likely to recognise:

- long night shifts, with limited and inconsistent rest periods
- insufficient sleep in between or prior to shifts
- busy workload during shifts
- dietary and exercise factors, including alcohol use
- work–life balance including family and study commitments
- environmental factors related to rural areas and hot weather.

As most of these factors relate to both work and home life, the responsibility for optimally managing fatigue is shared between the individual and employer. When adopting an HF/E approach, some elements of the pre-hospital work system that can be designed to mitigate fatigue are as follows:

- changes to shifts patterns
- shorter duration of shifts
- scheduled breaks
- education and resources related to fatigue management
- monitoring of fatigue levels.

(Ramey et al, 2019)

Shift working is often recognised to be a main contributory factor related to fatigue, therefore traditional focus in ambulance services has been to reduce shift length time and ensure enough rest between shifts (Ramey et al, 2019). It is important to note that there is not likely to be a perfect shift pattern that completely mitigates against worker fatigue. However, it is suggested that direction (morning to evening to night) and speed (of shift rotation, time of shift change, time off in between shifts and shift duration) are some principles that can be considered to synchronise circadian rhythms with shift patterns (Flin et al, 2008).

Education of staff about the effects of fatigue on performance (in a similar way to stress awareness) would also be helpful. With increased knowledge and understanding, ambulance clinicians can play their part in managing fatigue.

Chapter 7 – Well-Being of the Paramedic

Consideration of factors outside of work that would help manage fatigue and subsequently well-being, performance and safety include commuting arrangements after nightshifts and adjusting home arrangements to optimise good sleep hygiene (length and quality of sleep through attention to room temperature, intake of food, caffeine and alcohol, and screen time).

Summary

Optimising the well-being of workers in a system is not only a key objective of the discipline of HF/E but it is vitally important to a healthy workplace and creating a positive, supportive and engaging occupational culture. Understanding how the interacting elements of the work system affect well-being, how well-being and system performance are intertwined and how to recognise when well-being is affected, are absolutely fundamental. While various approaches may be taken to enhance the holistic experience of work, the HF/E approach specifically promotes a perhaps less acknowledged perspective that upholds design of the interactions within the work system as a way to optimise well-being. Within the field of paramedicine, this is certainly a relatively new way of viewing work, particularly in terms of processes and systems, which if not understood may adversely influence organisations and individual employees, and ultimately patient care. However, insightful knowledge, developed awareness and sustained commitment to humanise the workplace can only lead to more positive outcomes.

References

Aasa, U. et al. (2005). Work-related psychosocial factors, worry about work conditions, and health complaints among female and male ambulance personnel. *Scandinavian Journal of Caring Sciences*. 19: 251–258.

Asbury, E. et al. (2018). IPAWS: The International Paramedic Anxiety Wellbeing and Stress Study. *Emergency Medicine Australasia*. 30(1): 132.

Association of Ambulance Chief Executives (AACE) (2018a). Employee Mental Health Strategy Guidance [online]. Available from: https://www.nhsemployers.org/-/media/Employers/Documents/Ambulance-workforce/AACE-Employee-Mental-Health-Strategy-Guidance.pdf

Association of Ambulance Chief Executives (AACE) (2018b). Project A – Improving NHS Ambulance Services, Launch event London 28th June 2018 [online]. Available from: https://aace.org.uk/wp-content/uploads/2018/07/Improving-ambulance-services-28-June-2018.pdf

Bennett, P. et al. (2005). Associations between organisational and incident factors and emotional distress in emergency ambulance personnel. *British Journal of Clinical Psychology*. 44: 215–226.

Black, C. (2012). Work, health and wellbeing. *Safety and Health at Work*. 3(4): 241–242.

Bounds, R. (2006). Factors affecting perceived stress in pre-hospital emergency medical services. *Californian Journal of Health Promotion*. 4(2): 113–131.

Carayon, P. et al. (2014a). Human factors systems approach to healthcare quality and patient safety. *Applied Ergonomics*. 45(1): 14–25.

Carayon, P., Xie, A., Kianfar, S. (2014b). Human factors and ergonomics as a patient safety practice. *BMJ Quality & Safety*. 23: 196–205.

Corman, M.K. (2017). Driving to work: The front seat work of paramedics to and from the scene. *Symbolic Interaction*. 41(3): 291–310.

References

Department of Health (2013). Wellbeing and health [online]. Available from: https://assets.publishing.service.gov.uk/government/uploads/system/uploads/attachment_data/file/225525/DH_wellbeing_health.PDF

Dul, J. et al. (2012). A strategy for human factors/ergonomics: Developing the discipline and profession. *Ergonomics*. 55(4): 377–395.

Flin, R., O'Connor, P., Crichton, M. (2008). *Safety at the Sharp End: A Guide to Non-Technical Skills*. Aldershot: Ashgate.

Granter, E. et al. (2019). Multiple dimensions of work intensity: Ambulance work as edgework. *Work, Employment and Society*. 33(2): 280–297.

Hancox, B. (2019). Paramedic Peer Support Programme. *Paramedic Insight*. 5(2): 6.

Health Education England (2019). NHS Staff and Learners' Mental Wellbeing Report: Mental Wellbeing Report [online]. Available from: https://www.hee.nhs.uk/our-work/mental-wellbeing-report

Health and Safety Executive (2019). Work-related stress and how to tackle it [online]. Available from: https://www.hse.gov.uk/stress/what-to-do.htm

Hird, K. et al. (2019). OP6 An investigation into suicide amongst ambulance service staff. *Emergency Medicine Journal*. 3(6): e3.

Javaid, M.U. et al. (2017). Human Factors in Context to Occupational Health and Wellbeing. In: *Handbook of Research on Organisational Culture and Diversity in the Modern Workplace*. Christiansen, B., Chandan, C.H. (eds). Hershey, PA: IGI Global.

Jenner, M. (2007). The psychological impact of responding to agricultural emergencies. *The Australian Journal of Emergency Management*. 22(2): 25–31.

Jonsson, A., Segesten, K. (2003). Daily stress and concept of self in Swedish ambulance personnel. *Prehospital & Disaster Medicine*. 19(3): 226–234.

Jurisova, E. (2016). Coping strategies and post-traumatic growth in paramedics: Moderating effect of specific self-efficacy and positive/negative affectivity. *Studia Psychologica*. 58(4): 259–275.

Kupriyanov, R., Zhdanov, R. (2014). The eustress concept: Problems and outlooks. *World Journal of Medical Sciences*. 11(2): 179–185.

Lazarus, R.S. (1993). From psychological stress to the emotions: A history of changing outlooks. In: Porter, L.W., Rosenzweig, M.R. (eds). *Annual Review of Psychology* (Vol. 44). Palo Alto, CA: Annual Reviews, pp. 1–21.

Maguire, B.J. et al. (2014). Occupational injury risk among Australian paramedics: An analysis of national data. *Medical Journal of Australia*. 200(8): 477–480.

Maslow, A.H. (1943). A theory of human motivation. *Psychological Review*. 50(4): 370–396.

Maslow, A.H. (1962). *Towards a Psychology of Being*. Princeton: D Van Nostrand Company.

McFarlane, A.C., Bryant, R.A. (2007). Post-traumatic stress disorder in occupational settings: Anticipating and managing the risk. *Occupational Medicine*. 57(6): 404-410.

McGowan, J., Gardner, G., Fletcher, R. (2006). Positive and negative affective outcomes of occupational stress. *New Zealand Journal of Psychology*. 35: 92–98.

MIND (2013). How to manage stress [online]. Available from: https://www.mind.org.uk/information-support/types-of-mental-health-problems/stress/what-is-stress/?gclid=EAIaIQobChMI6b24gtqE

MIND (2019). Wellbeing and mental health support in the emergency services: our learning and key recommendations for the sector [online]. Available from: https://www.mind.org.uk/media-a/4572/20046_mind-blue-light-programme-legacy-report-v12_online.pdf

Murray, E., Krahe, C., Goodsman D. (2018). Are medical students in prehospital care at risk of moral injury? *Emergency Medicine Journal*. 35: 590–594.

Chapter 7 – Well-Being of the Paramedic

National Operational Guidance (2017a). Causes of stress [online]. Available from: https://www.ukfrs.com/node/136/revisions/13998/view?bundle=section&id=17003&parent=17009

National Operational Guidance (2017b). Impact of stress [online]. Available from: https://www.ukfrs.com/node/136/revisions/13998/view?bundle=section&id=17005&parent=17009

NHS Digital (2019). Stress related sickness absence of paramedics in ambulance trusts, July 2017 to June 2018 [online]. Available from: https://digital.nhs.uk/data-and-information/find-data-and-publications/supplementary-information/2019-supplementary-information-files/staff-absence/stress-related-sickness-absence-of-paramedics-in-ambulance-trusts-july-2017-to-june-2018

NHS England (2018a). Lord Carter's review into unwarranted variation in NHS ambulance trusts [online]. Available from: https://www.england.nhs.uk/publication/lord-carters-review-into-unwarranted-variation-in-nhs-ambulance-trusts/

NHS England (2018b). Ambulance Response Programme Review [online]. Available from: https://www.england.nhs.uk/wp-content/uploads/2018/10/ambulance-response-programme-review.pdf

NHS England (2018c). NHS staff heath & wellbeing: CQUIN 2017–2019 Indicator 1 Implementation Support. Available from: https://www.england.nhs.uk/wp-content/uploads/2018/05/staff-health-wellbeing-cquin-2017-19-implementation-support.pdf

Paterson, J.L., Sofianopoulos, S., Williams, B. (2014). What paramedics think about when they think about fatigue: Contributing factors. *Emergency Medicine Australia*. 26: 139–144.

Patterson, P.D. et al. (2012). Association between poor sleep, fatigue, and safety outcomes in emergency medical services providers. *Prehospital Emergency Care*. 16(1): 86–97.

Petrie, K. et al. (2018a). Prevalence of PTSD and common mental disorders amongst ambulance personnel: A systematic review and meta-analysis. *Social Psychiatry Psychiatric Epidemiology*. 53(9): 897–909.

Petrie, K. et al. (2018b). The importance of manager support for the mental health and well-being of ambulance personnel. *PLOS ONE*. 13(5): e0197802. Available from: https://doi.org/10.1371/journal.pone.0197802

Public Health England (2019a). Workplace health: Applying all our health [online]. Available from: https://www.gov.uk/government/publications/workplace-health-applying-all-our-health/workplace-health-applying-all-our-health#core-principles-for-healthcare-professionals

Public Health England (2019b). Health matters: Health and work [online]. Available from: https://www.gov.uk/government/publications/health-matters-health-and-work/health-matters-health-and-work

Ramey, S. et al. (2019). Drowsy and dangerous? Fatigue in paramedics: an overview. *Irish Journal of Paramedicine*. 4(1): 1–9.

Reason, J. (2008). *The Human Contribution: Unsafe acts, accidents and heroic recoveries*. Farnham: Ashgate.

Regehr, C., Goldberg, G., Hughes, J. (2002). Exposure to human tragedy, empathy, and trauma in ambulance paramedics. *American Journal of Orthopsychology*. 72(4): 505–513.

Reid, J., Bromiley, M. (2012). Clinical human factors: The need to speak up to improve patient safety. *Nursing Standard*. 26(35): 35–40.

Selye, H. (1974). *Stress without Distress*. Philadelphia: Lippincott and Company.

Smith, H. (2018). The emergence of the tick box mental health culture [online]. Available from: https://www.thehrdirector.com/features/mental-health/emergence-tick-box-mental-health-culture/

Sterud, T. et al. (2011). A comparison of general and ambulance specific stressors: Predictors of job satisfaction and health problems in a nationwide one-year follow up study of Norwegian ambulance personnel. *Journal of Occupational Medicine and Toxicology*. 6(1): 1–9.

References

Stevenson, D., Farmer, P. (2017). Thriving at work. Available from: https://assets.publishing.service.gov.uk/government/uploads/system/uploads/attachment_data/file/658145/thriving-at-work-stevenson-farmer-review.pdf

Waddell, G., Burton, A.K. (2006). Is work good for your health and wellbeing? Available from: https://assets.publishing.service.gov.uk/government/uploads/system/uploads/attachment_data/file/209510/hwwb-is-work-good-for-you-exec-summ.pdf

Williams, R., Bisson, J., Kemp, V. (2014). Principles for responding to people's psychosocial and mental health needs after disasters [online]. Available from: https://www.apothecaries.org/wp-content/uploads/2018/05/OP94.pdf

World Health Organization (2009). Human factors in patient safety: Review of topics and tools [online]. Available from: https://www.who.int/patientsafety/research/methods_measures/human_factors/human_factors_review.pdf

World Health Organization (2013). The European Health Report 2012: Charting the way to well-being. WHO: Copenhagen [online]. Available from: http://www.euro.who.int/__data/assets/pdf_file/0004/197113/EHR2012-Eng.pdf

Yaribeygi, H. et al. (2017). The impact of stress on body function: A review. *Experimental and Clinical Sciences Journal* [online]. 16: 1057–1072. Available from: https://www.ncbi.nlm.nih.gov/pmc/articles/PMC5579396/

Chapter 8

Situation Awareness and Decision Making

Ben Shippey and Gary Rutherford

In this chapter:
- An introduction to non-technical skills
- Gaining and maintaining individual situation awareness in pre-hospital care
- Paramedic decision making in complex systems

Non-Technical Skills

Paramedics use a wide range of technical skills such as airway management, vascular access, medicine administration, wound management and fracture immobilisation. It is increasingly recognised that a paramedic's performance and well-being can benefit from understanding and applying non-technical skills in addition to their technical skills and knowledge. Non-technical skills are 'the cognitive and social skills that complement a worker's technical skills' (Flin et al, 2008), and they facilitate 'safe, effective and efficient task performance' (College of Paramedics, 2017).

'Non-technical skills' is an area of HF/E which is of particular interest to frontline professionals, as it helps them to understand their own performance and limitations. As this aspect of HF/E is concerned with cognitive functions, cognitive systems, behaviours and skills of individuals, it may be helpful to see it as 'factors of humans': you might want to refer back to Chapter 2. This suggestion may help to understand how non-technical skills are a small part of the overall discipline of HF/E, and address the common view in healthcare that non-technical skills 'are' human factors. Therefore, an HF/E approach would consider non-technical skills in the context of how they are relevant to the design of the work system, i.e. how the system can be designed to facilitate best performance and optimise non-technical skills.

The role that non-technical skills have in flight safety is established within the aviation industry, with weak non-technical skills identified as being contributing factors in the majority of fatal aviation incidents (Civil Aviation Authority, 2013).

Chapter 8 – Situation Awareness and Decision Making

As discussed in Chapter 2, significant aviation incidents in the 1970s led to the development of Crew Resource Management (CRM) training courses and non-technical skills assessment frameworks (NOTECHS), to educate, assess and provide feedback on the behaviours of aircrew. CRM and TRM (Team Resource Management) training can help people gain insight into their behaviours and influence them to change those behaviours to support effective team performance (Jégoux, 2018). If non-technical skills training is designed using HF/E approaches and becomes sufficiently established, a 'critical mass' will be reached and widespread implementation of optimal non-technical skills in daily practice can be achieved, improving the work system and the interactions within it.

Describing and quantifying non-technical skills can be challenging, but non-technical skills assessment tools (also referred to as behavioural marker systems) have been developed to observe and measure performance in a range of clinical fields. Examples of these include: ANTS (anaesthetists' non-technical skills), NOTSS (non-technical skills for surgeons) and SPLINTS (scrub practitioners' list of intraoperative non-technical skills). Non-technical skills related to paramedic practice are not well described in literature and a paramedic profession-specific behavioural marker system does not yet exist.

We should be clear that the behaviour is *not* the skill: the behaviour is what we observe that allows us to make inferences about the skills that are being performed. Although paramedics' non-technical skills are likely to be similar to those in other healthcare disciplines, we should be cautious about simply applying or adapting other professions' frameworks to paramedic practice without specific research (Shields and Flin, 2013), and the behaviours that we might observe that would allow us to describe the non-technical skills of paramedics will of course be different. The non-technical skills that are identified in these other disciplines that could be applicable and practised by paramedics are listed below, although Bennett et al (2020) suggest that there may be as many as 26 paramedic non-technical skills worthy of future consideration and research:

- situation awareness
- decision making
- team working
- leadership
- communication
- task management.

Individual situation awareness and decision making will be discussed in this chapter, with Chapter 9 considering shared situation awareness and teamwork (incorporating leadership, communication and task management). Non-technical skills related to human performance of tasks are informed by some theories of psychology. Therefore, if paramedic performance within the pre-hospital system is to be optimised, it will be useful to have some understanding of the psychological processes that are used, the limitations of those processes, and some routes around the pitfalls that can lead to undesired outcomes.

Situation Awareness and Decision Making

Making decisions is an activity that all ambulance clinicians will recognise as an integral part of their clinical practice. Those decisions are changing in response to shifts in patient demographics and patterns of disease (Collen, 2017). Societies' experiences and expectations of the paramedic profession have altered since its inception and the need for ambulance clinicians to make increasingly complex decisions regarding patient triage, treatment and referral have become vital to improving patient outcomes and safety.

Decisions are based on an understanding of the situation that is encountered. The ability of humans to appreciate, assimilate and make meaning from vast amounts of data, and use the interpretation that is subsequently generated to make (sometimes) rapid, informed decisions and enact them is an impressive process. The result of that interpretation is called 'situation awareness', which may be a term that is not as well recognised or understood as decision making; there is certainly a lack of literature regarding situation awareness in paramedic practice (Hunter et al, 2019).

Situation Awareness

Situation awareness encompasses the process by which we perceive stimuli (for example, sounds, visual images, smells), make meaning from those inputs, and then project forward to generate an expectation of what we anticipate will happen next. To generate optimal situation awareness, an individual needs to gather enough information from the environment to form an accurate 'mental model' of the situation (Fortune et al, 2013). Situation awareness is particularly pertinent to decision making in dynamic situations (Endsley, 1995), which is of course relevant to ambulance clinicians working in the ever-changing environment of pre-hospital care.

Although there is not a universally agreed definition of situation awareness (Stanton et al, 2017), there are several suggestions. It has been described as simply 'knowing what is going on around you', where individuals continuously monitor the surrounding environment for things that are happening or changing (Flin et al, 2008). Others suggest that situation awareness is as much about anticipating future events as it is about understanding the current situation (Golightly, 2015). We will focus on the definition proposed by Endsley (1995) which combines elements of both, and aligns to her model:

> ... the **perception** of the elements in the environment within a volume of time and space, the **comprehension** of their meaning and the **projection** of their status in the near future.

> *Mental model – a strongly debated concept, with no agreed definition. Generally considered to be a picture in the mind of the current situation, although it may not be accurate or shared with others.*

Chapter 8 – Situation Awareness and Decision Making

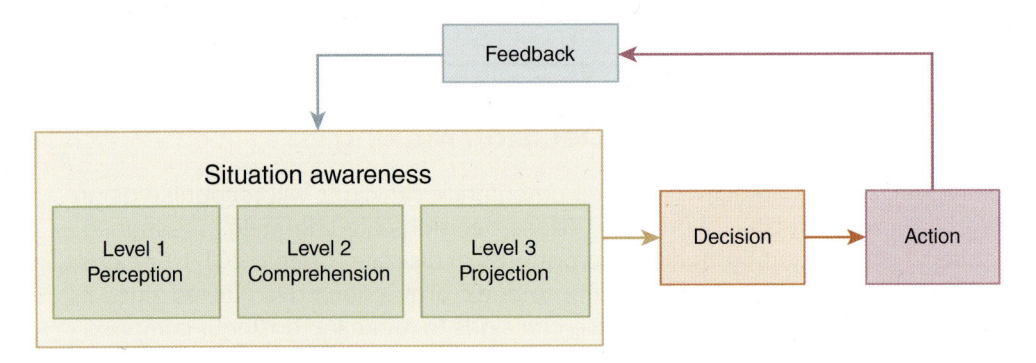

Figure 8.1 – Situation awareness and decision making in Endsley's model of situation awareness

Endsley's (1995) three-level model of situation awareness (Figure 8.1) illustrates how situation awareness and decision making are linked. Crucially, it presents development of situation awareness as a process that occurs prior to decision making.

There is debate regarding the models and cognitive processes that underpin situation awareness (Flin et al, 2008). Endsley's model has been challenged as being too focused on the psychology of the individual and not sufficiently reflecting the complexity of how situation awareness is influenced by the individuals' interaction with other elements (for example, technology) of a system (Stanton et al 2010, 2017). Despite this, it is a model that is useful in introducing a complex cognitive skill such as situation awareness, and it is proposed as the most appropriate framework to apply to paramedic practice (Hunter et al, 2020).

Three Levels of Situation Awareness

In Endsley's model of situation awareness, the three levels (Figure 8.2) are based on the perception, comprehension and projection elements highlighted in the definition. These are central to this model and are also often described as 'What?', 'So what?' and 'Now what?'

Although each level is illustrated in a linear format, the stages of situation awareness processes are often not sequential. Lauria et al (2019) describe how it is a 'cyclic

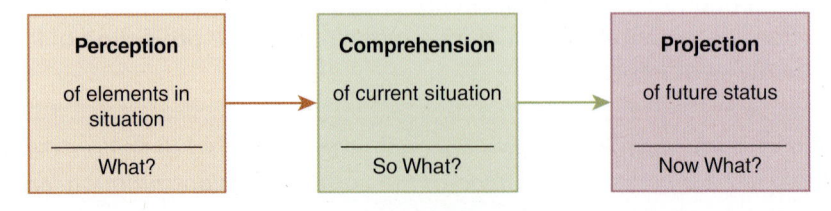

Figure 8.2 – Three levels of situation awareness

and dynamic' process, which can involve individuals constantly re-evaluating the situation. Therefore, a paramedic can go through this process multiple times, or restart the process before completion, as new information becomes available or more relevant. For example, during emergency response driving, information being presented and available can change quickly, requiring the ambulance crew to perceive new information that may affect understanding and projection. These levels are explored in more detail below.

Level 1 – Perception (What?)

This level of situation awareness is related to how humans perceive information from the environment. The brain is constantly receiving sensory inputs via our senses of sight, hearing, touch, taste and smell. However, we do not consciously appreciate all these inputs as there are often too many to process. The way in which an individual 'tunes in' to some of those inputs and (consciously and unconsciously) disregards others is called 'attention'. It is this selective attention process that forms the basis for situation awareness (Flin et al, 2008).

When a paramedic arrives 'on scene' at an incident or call, they are exposed to a significant number of sensory inputs, and are faced with the challenge of identifying which ones need attention. Flin et al (2008) specifically suggest that emergency service workers particularly rely on these perceptual skills.

Attention is a limited resource and it can be difficult for a person to concentrate on more than one thing at a time. Therefore, it can be easy to overlook information that is readily available. Failure to perceive information is a common reason for not achieving optimal situation awareness. The shortcomings of our attention can be exposed and demonstrated in a few ways:

- **Tunnel vision:** Where we can become so focused on a task, such as vascular cannulation, that we fail to notice other information such as a colleague speaking to us or the monitor alarming. Auditory information is easily shut out by the brain.

- **Inattentional blindness:** When we are not aware of something in our visual field as our attention is directed elsewhere within that field. This has been demonstrated in experiments, the most famous being when participants fail to notice a person in a gorilla suit walking among other people playing basketball. This is due to attention being directed to the other people throwing the basketball. Search online for 'The Invisible Gorilla' or 'The Monkey Business Illusion' to watch demonstrations of inattentional blindness.

- **Change blindness:** In change blindness we fail to notice the difference in a change between the current and previous state. This is subtly different to inattentional blindness. Search online for 'The Door Study' or 'Simons and Levin, Change Blindness' to watch experiments of how people fail to notice that the person they are speaking to has changed.

Chapter 8 – Situation Awareness and Decision Making

Level 2 – Comprehension (So What?)

Level 2 situation awareness involves the individual making sense of the sensory data that has been perceived to form an understanding of the situation and generate a mental model of what is happening. Comprehension is based on correctly perceiving the information, retaining it in short-term memory (can also be called working memory), in addition to retrieving knowledge from long-term memory (Flin et al, 2008). Therefore, if information has not been perceived correctly or the ambulance clinician does not have the required experience or knowledge, an incorrect mental model can be formed, which may have implications for future decision making and patient safety.

This perception–comprehension information processing is fallible, and this can be demonstrated by considering some well-known 'illusions'. When most people view the image in Figure 8.3, they perceive that the top horizontal line is longer than the bottom one. Even once you know that the lines are the same length (they are!), you will still likely perceive that the top one is longer than the bottom one.

In the image in Figure 8.4, it can be hard to convince the brain that the horizontal lines are all parallel.

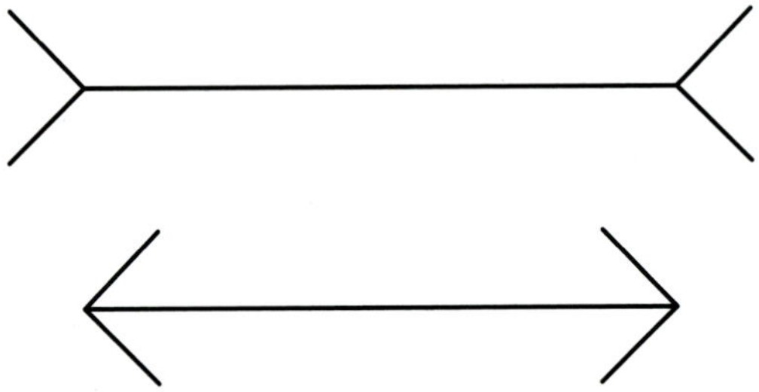

Figure 8.3 – Müller-Lyer illusion
Source: Based on Müller-Lyer (1889)

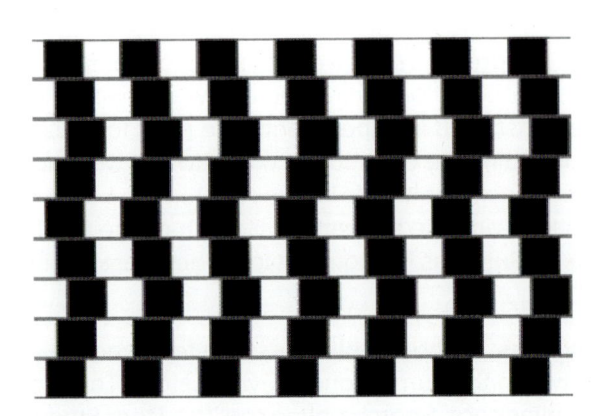

Figure 8.4 – Café Wall illusion
Source: Based on Gregory and Heard (1979); Image from Fibonacci via Wikimedia Commons (CC BY-SA 3.0)

No one fully knows how optical illusions work and different illusions probably trick the brain in different ways. However, it is believed that the effects of colour and light, and arrangement of patterns create a difference between reality and perception that is misleading to our brains. The brain can often attempt to take a short cut to interpret information and these images can expose this process. Therefore, when operating in the real world, it is not beyond the realms of possibility that something could be 'seen' but misinterpreted by the brain.

Level 3 – Projection (Now What?)

The 'projection of future status' stage is about using the gained understanding and mental model from levels 1 and 2 to consider and anticipate what is going to happen in the immediate future, i.e. 'if this situation continues, then x will likely happen'. Projection is not the same as decision making – it is the process of thinking ahead that leads into making a decision. Flin et al (2008) state that this stage of situation awareness is crucial in dynamic environments where conditions are continually changing.

Examples of Situation Awareness

Look at the picture in Figure 8.5, imagining that you are responding to an emergency in an ambulance vehicle, and think what you would do.

You probably decided to apply or at least cover the brakes and arriving at that decision likely took less than a second to make. It was gaining appropriate situation awareness that lead to that decision. If we apply Endsley's model we can demonstrate and analyse each stage further:

- What do you **see**?
- What is that likely to **mean**?
- What might **happen** next?

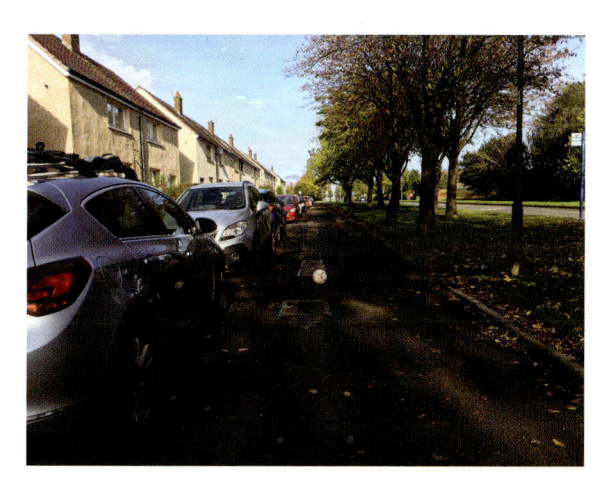

Figure 8.5 – What would you do?
Source: Gary Rutherford

Chapter 8 – Situation Awareness and Decision Making

You see a ball, bouncing out from between two parked cars. This is your *perception* (actually, your perception is of a pattern of white and black shapes which you recognise as a 'ball', but for the sake of simplicity, we'll say that you perceive a ball). Footballs are often associated with children and although you can't actually see a child, you generate *understanding* that 'there is probably a child, that I can't see because of the cars, that is playing with that football'. You then think ahead, using previous experience and understanding of how situations such as this might develop, you *project* forwards into the future, and anticipate that the child, probably without looking for traffic, will run out from between the parked cars, and before you've even realised it, your foot is over the brake pedal.

Pre-Hospital Examples

We can also apply the three-stage model to examples from pre-hospital clinical care in Figures 8.6 and 8.7.

Example 1: Low Saturations

You are assessing a patient who has become acutely unwell at home. Your colleague attaches the pulse oximeter and you notice a low reading of 89%. You may also notice the monitor alarm which is designed to bring this to your attention.

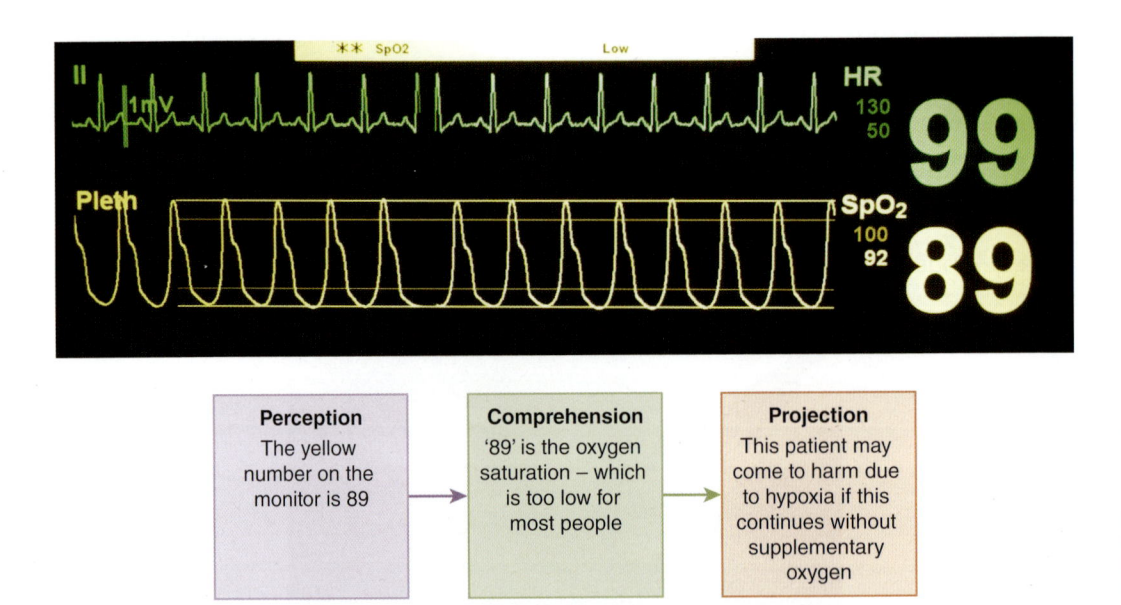

Perception	Comprehension	Projection
The yellow number on the monitor is 89	'89' is the oxygen saturation – which is too low for most people	This patient may come to harm due to hypoxia if this continues without supplementary oxygen

Figure 8.6 – Low oxygen saturations

Example 2: Road Traffic Collision

You are attending to a road traffic collision which is reported to be a car versus a pedestrian. On arrival you see that an adult appears to have been knocked down near a pedestrian crossing.

The Role of Memory in Situation Awareness

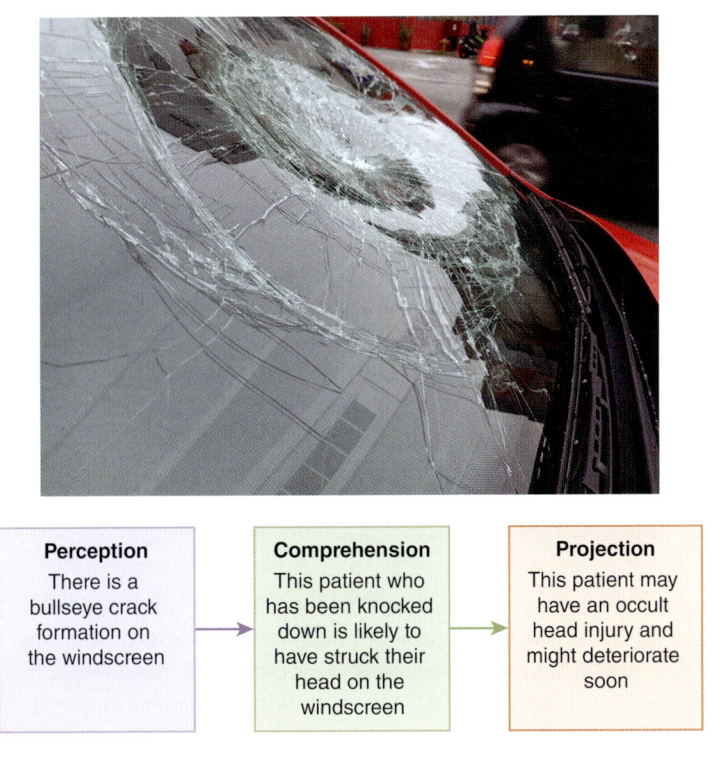

Perception	Comprehension	Projection
There is a bullseye crack formation on the windscreen	This patient who has been knocked down is likely to have struck their head on the windscreen	This patient may have an occult head injury and might deteriorate soon

Figure 8.7 – Road traffic collision
Source: Ummi Hassian / Shutterstock

The Role of Memory in Situation Awareness

The brain has two main memory stores – working memory (also called short-term memory) and long-term memory, and these memory processes are key to situation awareness and decision making (Endsley, 1995). It is the working memory that initially receives the sensory input and retains it for a short period of time. Working memory has a limited capacity and is very susceptible to losing information if other sensory inputs are received while trying to retain the initial inputs. An example is trying to remember a telephone number that you have just been told. You are likely to 'chunk' the number into three or four easier-to-retain smaller numbers and repeat it to ensure it is retained for longer. However, if another prominent stimulus is received or distraction occurs, it is likely that the number will be forgotten. In hospital, when clinicians are preparing and administering medication, they are recommended to wear coloured aprons or tabards to identify that they should not be distracted. This is to reduce medication errors associated with interrupting working memory processes (Grissinger, 2015).

Long-term memory is the store for all the information an individual has received throughout their lifetime. In relation to situation awareness, information can be retrieved from long-term memory to help generate understanding of the situation. This is important to situation awareness because it may be difficult to retain a large number of different perceptions in short-term memory long enough to

Chapter 8 – Situation Awareness and Decision Making

develop Level 1 situation awareness. And the retrieval of previous knowledge and experience from long-term memory is useful to the development of Level 2 and 3 situation awareness.

Maintaining Situation Awareness

The Civil Aviation Authority (CAA) identify 'loss of situation awareness' as a contributing factor in a high proportion of aviation incidents, although they also urge caution in attributing this as the 'cause' and recommend that accident reviews go beyond this (CAA, 2016). It is important to ensure that 'not gaining situation awareness', or 'losing situation awareness', does not just become another way of saying 'human error'. The concept of situation awareness is criticised by some: Sidney Dekker suggests that hindsight analysis of an incident always shows that 'there was more in the world than there was in the mind' (Dekker, 2015). The challenge is to identify why individuals were not aware of something and design the work system to maximise situation awareness.

Pilots who have formed a mental model that is different to reality are said to have lost situation awareness, although they are unlikely to be aware of this and continue to feel normal (CAA, 2016). Situation awareness can be lost, then regained, with the pilot being unaware that this has occurred. This highlights some significant challenges in self-identifying when situation awareness may be affected or suboptimal. A number of signs or indications that situation awareness is being affected are proposed (Flin et al, 2008; CAA, 2016), although it can be challenging to recognise them in yourself in 'real time'.

Possible signs that your situation awareness might be affected are:

- ambiguity – when information from two or more sources does not agree
- fixation – focusing on one thing to the exclusion of other information
- confusion – uncertainty or bafflement about a situation (often accompanied by anxiety or psychological discomfort)
- failure to maintain critical tasks
- failure to meet an expected target
- inability to resolve discrepancies with contradictory data or personal conflicts
- not communicating effectively or team members go 'heads down'.

Specific things can be done to minimise the risk of reduced situation awareness in individuals and teams. Pre-task briefings can be held, for planned events, in which the expectations, risks and contingencies that occur at different stages or phases can be defined. The 'sterile cockpit' concept adopted from aviation can be utilised, where communication is restricted to clinical procedure and safety matters only during crucial periods of critical care, and where interruptions are only permitted if they relate to immediate situation safety concerns.

There are both active and passive processes that can influence situation awareness in critical care transport (Lauria et al, 2019). An example of a passive element that could enhance situation awareness is a monitor alarm which can be designed or set to maximise the perception of information related to a change in patient condition. Active processes are individual behaviours of deliberate focus and scanning or monitoring of the environment, monitors or clinical features, in order to identify a problem at an early stage. Using this method, the clinician can perform a practised sequence of checks of key features to minimise the risk that information is not perceived.

It would be unreasonable to suggest that paramedics can always maintain optimal situation awareness, due to the amount of sensory information that is available and changing, in addition to the effort and attention that would be required to actively scan and consider one's own situation awareness status. However, having an understanding of situation awareness and how it can become affected may encourage individuals to take a moment (stepping back from the scene or patient if appropriate) and ask themselves the following:

- Am I aware of what is going on around me?
- Are things happening as they are supposed to be happening?
- If not, why not?
- If things go wrong, what is the plan?
- Are other members of my team 'on the same page'? I.e. do we have a shared mental model?

Making Decisions

Decisions can be made in several ways, and depending on the circumstances, different techniques are used (Flin et al, 2008). Paramedics often work in dynamic environments where the conditions and patient presentation can be variable and unpredictable, and these factors make paramedic decision making unique from other healthcare professionals (Jensen et al, 2016). In this dynamic world, a single approach to decision making is likely to be limiting, therefore it will be helpful to explore different decision-making theories and models, and relate each to paramedic practice.

It is important to note that clinicians don't always consciously choose which method of decision making is appropriate for the situation, although having an increased awareness and understanding of decision-making theories may help to recognise situations where the various decision-making strategies could be more (or less) useful.

Evolution of Decision Making

Decision-making theories have evolved from 'classical decision theory' in the 1950s, where it was proposed that people made rational decisions by recognising there is a

Chapter 8 – Situation Awareness and Decision Making

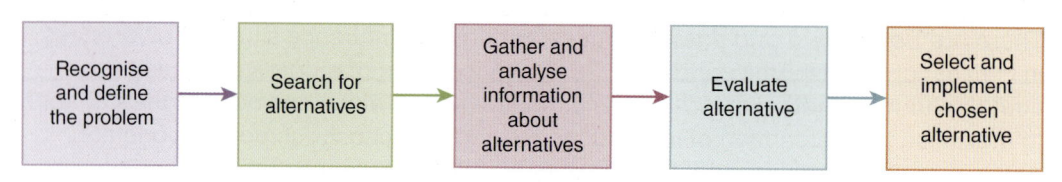

Recognise and define the problem → Search for alternatives → Gather and analyse information about alternatives → Evaluate alternative → Select and implement chosen alternative

Figure 8.8 – Rational model of decision making
Source: Created by Scott MacKenzie; based on Buchanan and Huczynski (2019)

problem, then taking a step-wise approach to identify and evaluate options, before choosing the most optimal one (Figure 8.8). However, this approach was developed in relation to the social science of economics and 'assumes that decision makers are objective, have complete information and consider all possible alternatives and their consequences before selecting the optimal solution' (Buchanan and Huczynski, 2019).

This might be how some people think that they would choose a new car, or buy a house, and while this is one way in which decisions can be made, you may recognise that some of the decisions that you make (like the decision to apply the brakes in the example earlier) are not made on the basis of generating a long list of options. They simply 'happen', particularly when decisions need to be made quickly.

By the late 1980s, it was acknowledged that this classical theory of rational decision making was not typically the way that people made decisions in the 'real world' (Klein, 2008). Through observing and interviewing decision makers in aviation, military and emergency services, a new concept of 'naturalistic decision making' theory emerged (Flin et al, 2008). This theory contrasts with classical theory by suggesting that decisions are not made by rational analysis and comparison of options. Instead, decision makers used prior experiences to rapidly categorise situations, particularly in dynamic environments where there may be competing goals and time pressure (Klein, 2008). One model of naturalistic decision making is 'recognition-primed' decision making, which is discussed later in the chapter.

System 1 and System 2

Dual Process Theory is a leading explanation of how decision making occurs (Jensen et al, 2016), adopting themes from both classical and naturalistic theories. The dual process allows decisions to occur in response to two systems in the mind – System 1 and System 2, also known as 'thinking fast' and 'thinking slow', respectively. System 1 'operates automatically and quickly, with little or no effort and no sense of voluntary control' (thinking fast), whereas System 2 'allocates attention to the effortful mental activities that demand it' (thinking slow) (Kahneman, 2012).

System 1

System 1 is informed by experiences and knowledge to generate rapid, effortless patterns. Thinking and decision making using this mode occurs intuitively thousands of times each day and deals with the majority of everyday thinking.

Heuristics – cognitive short cuts, abbreviated ways of thinking. 'Seen this many times' (Croskerry et al, 2013).

Simple questions such as 'what is the capital of France?' and 'what is the answer to 2 + 2 = ?' demonstrate this involuntary mode of thinking, where the answer can almost not be avoided from entering our thoughts, if we have the knowledge (Kahneman, 2012). This spontaneous way of making a decision can also be characterised by a predominant use of 'heuristics', is context-dependent and highly susceptible to biases (see below) or influences that may not be relevant to the problem at hand. System 1 thinking is frugal, in terms of its cognitive demand, and occurs very quickly. While it is often correct, it can be prone to error (Croskerry et al, 2013). Thinking fast to make decisions therefore has some parallels with the naturalistic decision-making theory.

System 2

In contrast, System 2 requires more cognitive effort, and is usually engaged when the problem at hand does not readily 'match' an easily found solution, i.e. System 1 is unable to make sense of the situation. The process is characterised by a methodical approach to elaborating and understanding the facts of the problem, and recalling, or generating, a decision that System 1 had difficulty doing, but at the cost of time and effort. People mostly consider themselves as predominantly System 2 thinkers and decision makers, however the reality is that System 1 is the most dominant way of thinking (Kahneman, 2012). We spend most of our daily activities (up to 95% of our time) in the intuitive mode of System 1 (Croskerry et al, 2013).

System 2 is normally in a 'low-effort mode' and only 'takes over' when things get difficult for System 1. In contrast to the 2 + 2 =? question that System 1 found easy, $17 \times 24 = ?$ causes System 1 some difficulty to intuitively provide a quick correct answer, and System 2 steps in to calculate the answer. It is important to appreciate that these two systems do not act independently, rather they are both active when we are awake and interact with each other depending on the situation.

It is possible, although challenging, to influence the mode of decision making that is appropriate to the situation that ambulance clinicians are involved with, provided that we are aware of the cognitive processes being used to generate decisions. This may involve recognising moments when we should attempt to slow down to gather more information and consider options. The process of being aware of the way in which we are thinking is called 'metacognition', and is also helpful in avoiding bias.

Bias

Biases in decision making are essentially subconscious errors where judgement has been unduly influenced by other factors (Croskerry et al, 2013). Due to the speed and use of heuristics in System 1 thinking, this method is very susceptible to bias.

Understanding the influence of individual biases is an important first step for the clinician to start to identify the unconscious influencers upon their decision making in clinical practice. There are many different biases which can influence decision making in paramedic practice (Collen, 2017). The key ones to note are outlined in Table 8.1.

Table 8.1 – Common cognitive biases

Bias	Description
Priming effect	Being recently exposed to something that subconsciously influences later decisions
Anchoring bias	Focusing and relying too heavily on an initial piece of information and failing to adjust in light of further and later information
Availability bias	Making a decision based on availability of recent memories or experience of making a similar decision
Confirmation bias	Looking for and favouring further information to support an earlier decision, while subconsciously discounting other information that doesn't support it

Source: Based on Hearns, 2019.

Paramedic Decision Making

Literature related to studies specifically looking at decision making by paramedics is limited (Jensen et al, 2016; Perona et al, 2019). However, themes of System 1 and System 2 thinking are evident. Experienced paramedics probably use intuition (System 1) frequently, while those who have recently completed training and education may be more inclined to use analytical (System 2) hypothetico-deductive methods (Ryan and Halliwell, 2012). Both experienced and student paramedics *believe* that they use rational thinking and decision making more than relying upon their past experiences (Jensen et al, 2016), which may support Kahneman's observations about the incorrect belief that System 2 is used more frequently than System 1.

Model of Decision Making

A model of decision making that may well incorporate all these theories of thinking and decision making, while also highlighting the benefits and limitations of each, is proposed by Flin et al (2008) (Figure 8.9). This model suggests that there are four likely processes for making a decision, each with the possibility of being adopted by paramedics depending on the circumstances, with the level of risk and available

Model of Decision Making

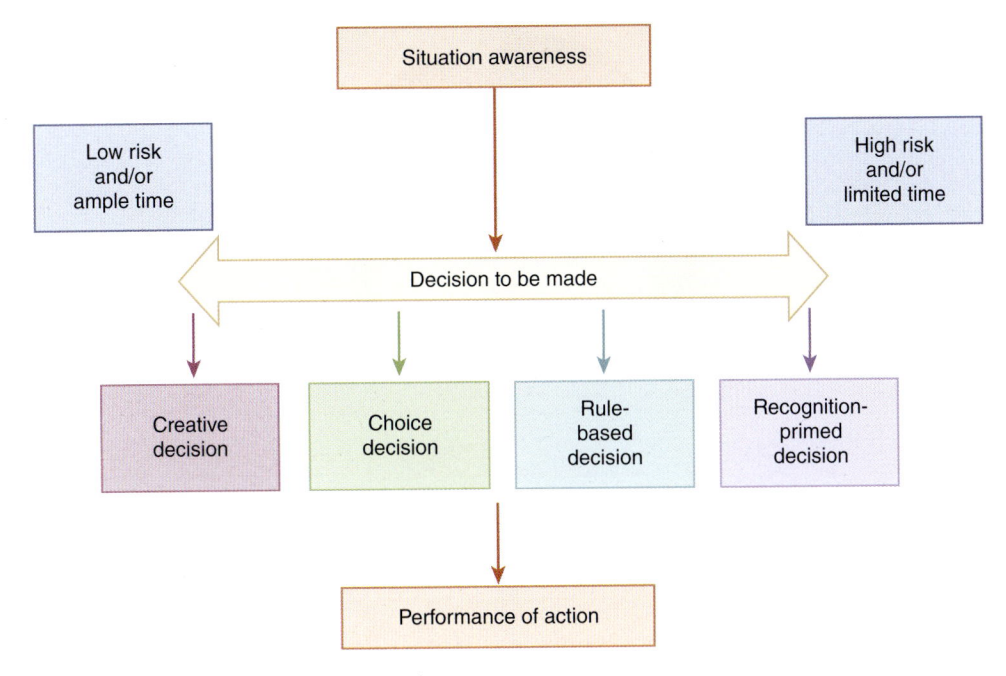

Figure 8.9 – Model of decision making
Source: Based on Flin et al (2008)

time as the main influencers of which strategy is applied. These decision-making processes are:

- recognition-primed
- rule-based
- choice
- creative.

Recognition-Primed Decision Making

Recognition-primed decision making (also called 'intuitive' decision making) is a model of naturalistic decision-making theory, where people with appropriate knowledge use experience to recognise patterns, and mental simulation of how things 'would play out', to initiate an action (Klein, 2008). This model was proposed after observation and interviews of US firefighter commanders in relation to recent challenging incidents where they had made crucial decisions. It seems that the decisions they made did not align with classical theories, and that recognition-primed type processes were observable in 80–90% of decisions. Instead of comparing multiple options concurrently and choosing an optimal one, fire commanders would generate and evaluate a single acceptable option based on patterns that they had used previously. This is often described as 'having a gut feeling', and usually happens quickly and with limited conscious control or awareness. This model incorporates aspects of both System 1 thinking (pattern recognition) and System 2

Chapter 8 – Situation Awareness and Decision Making

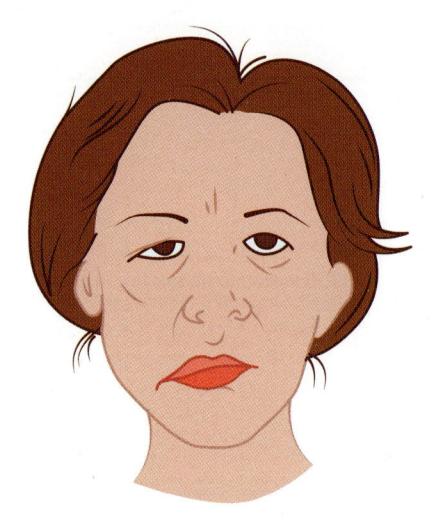

Figure 8.10 – Signs of a possible stroke

thinking (mental simulation) (Klein, 2008). Key to the understanding of recognition-primed decision making is that focus is on understanding and defining the situation at hand rather than generating multiple options (Flin et al, 2008), and that the response generated relies significantly on our previous experiences of similar situations and rapid retrieval of information from our long-term memory. While the option that we select may not necessarily be the best option, it will usually result in progress towards an acceptable goal.

Look at the face of the person in Figure 8.10. You will notice that they have drooping on the right side of their face, which started 30 minutes ago along with slurred speech. You are likely to recognise this pattern of clinical signs as a possible acute stroke. Your gut feeling or intuition may lead you to make a rapid decision to initiate timely extrication and transport to an appropriate hospital, and this decision may be reached quicker if you have significant knowledge and experience related to the management of previous patients experiencing a stroke. One advantage of recognition-primed decision making is that it requires very little cognitive effort, therefore can be done quickly, making it useful in time-critical situations. However, recognition-primed decision making is particularly susceptible to confirmation bias (Flin et al, 2008), and erroneous decisions can easily be made. In this example, you have made an acceptable decision to transport the patient to the correct hospital quickly, but if (due to lack of knowledge or previous experience) you fail to consider other stroke-mimic conditions, your decision making could be viewed retrospectively as suboptimal. Recognising that your assessment is intuitive, and actively reconsidering it if subsequent developments don't 'fit' with your decision, will help mitigate against confirmation bias.

Experience and intuition are very useful in certain circumstances, although one should be cautious in situations where decisions cannot be 'remade' (Collen, 2017). For example, recognition-primed decision making would not be an ideal approach when deciding to administer a medicine by the intravenous route. A more structured and slower method of decision making would be more suitable in order to ensure patient safety.

Rule-Based Decision Making

In some situations, it is more appropriate to make decisions using rules that have been determined in advance, and it would be reasonable to suggest that paramedic practice is strongly influenced by 'rules'. An example is the *JRCALC Clinical Guidelines* reference edition (JRCALC, 2019) which has over 600 pages of guidance, protocols and procedures designed to support and guide clinicians' decision-making processes. Although the guidelines come with a disclaimer that they are 'advisory', it would be fair to say that they are considered clinical rules, where a strong rationale would be required if they were not applied.

Rule-based decision making involves 'identifying the situation encountered and remembering or looking up in a manual the rule or procedure that applies' (Flin et al, 2008). Accurately defining the situation is key, as applying the wrong rule may compromise the outcome. The process of looking up rules requires more cognitive effort (utilising System 2) and is a method often utilised by novices, who are learning the rules. More experienced clinicians can also make rule-based decisions, although this can often occur without looking the rule up, particularly if the rule being applied is one that they are very familiar with and have learned through repeated use. In this way it can be applied rapidly, with little cognitive effort, almost becoming intuitive (System 1). The experienced clinician may need to look up a rule if it is an infrequently applied one that has not been stored in long-term memory.

Finding the required rules can sometimes be a challenge in paramedic practice. Guidelines, protocols and standard operating procedures are proliferating rapidly and may not always be readily available. They are often stored on internal IT systems, desktop computers which have secure access and are not often well indexed, or on a variety of noticeboards in ambulance stations. There can also be an assumption that the protocols are correct, and kept up to date, which may not necessarily always be the case. A recent development in the UK is that all ambulance services have adopted use of the JRCALC app as a digital platform for ambulance clinicians to access the required most up-to-date national and local guidelines. This is a significant move away from pocketbooks, changing the interacting elements of this work system. The benefits of digital platforms and updates should be considered alongside the design of the app and availability of the device, to ensure it is easy for ambulance clinicians to access the required guidance when they need it. In demanding situations, utilisation of an effective guideline assists with 'cognitive offloading' and supports accurate decision making (Hearns, 2019), and can make it easier for the decision maker to justify their actions after the event.

In paramedic practice, perhaps the best known set of rules that are followed are those that govern the initial management of cardiac arrest (Figure 8.11). All that is required is to determine the absence of vital signs, after which the 'rules' should be applied. The series of actions have been agreed in advance by experts, with each

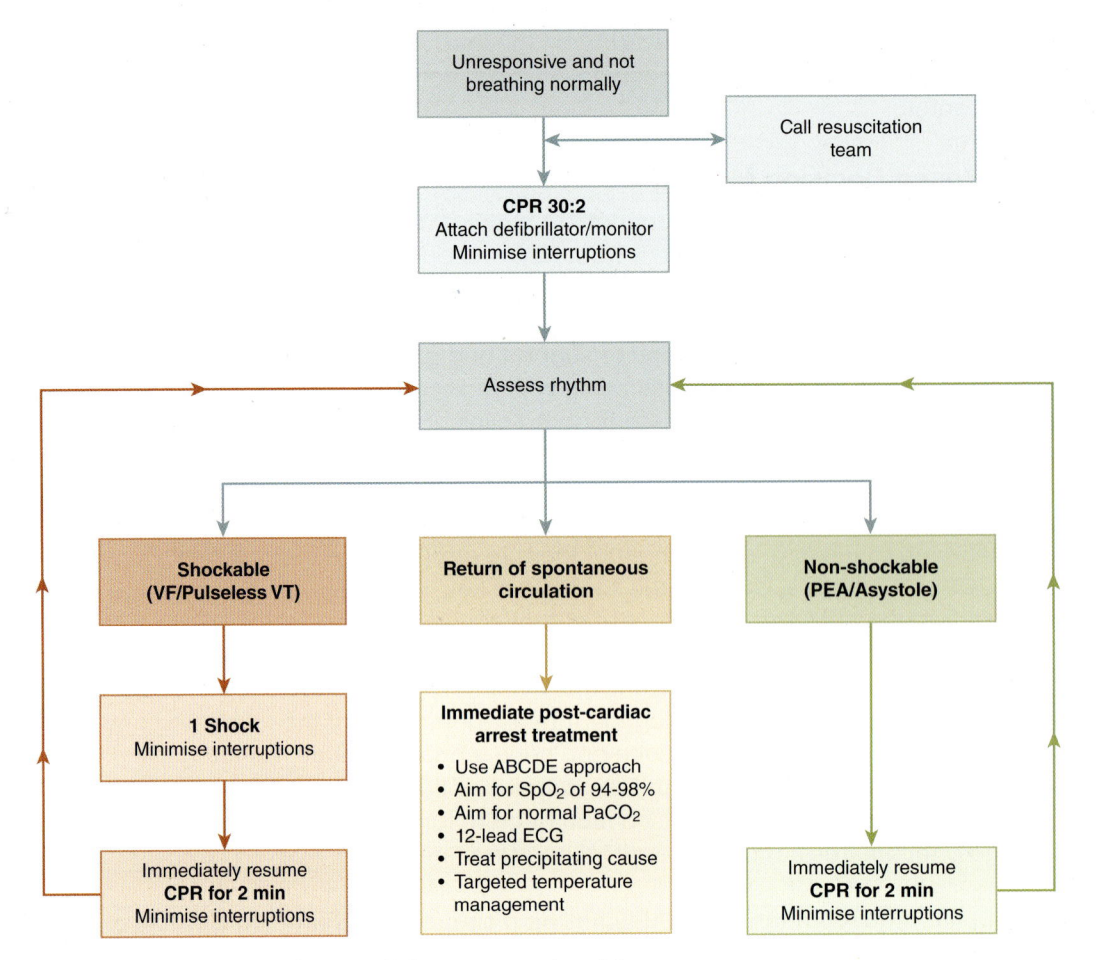

Chapter 8 – Situation Awareness and Decision Making

Figure 8.11 – Adult advanced life support algorithm
Source: Resuscitation Council (UK) (2015). Reproduced with permission.

subsequent decision to be made being determined by relatively straightforward assessments of responses to previous actions. Clinicians are not required to make many subjective judgements until the consideration of reversible causes, or deemed that it is appropriate to cease resuscitation.

Choice Decision Making

Choice decision-making methods (sometimes called analytical) originate from the classical decision-making theory discussed earlier. Options are considered and evaluated, with the optimal choice identified as the best to meet the needs of the situation. This type of analytical thinking is also associated with the hypothetico-deductive type decision making discussed by Collen (2017), where clinicians would form a possible hypothesis, then work through patient assessment processes to 'rule in' and 'rule out' other options and differential diagnoses. This would obviously take time, therefore may be a challenging process in a time-critical situation. This type of decision making aligns to System 2 ('thinking slow').

Model of Decision Making

Examples in pre-hospital care may be when considering analgesia, extrication or non-conveyance options in non-time-critical situations.

Creative Decision Making

Infrequently in pre-hospital care, the clinician may encounter a situation for which there are no predetermined 'rules', for which they have no previous experience or 'intuition', and where no favourable options can be identified through choice processes. In this situation, a more creative method of making decisions is needed. This requires a lot of cognitive effort and utilisation of System 2, to understand the situation based on our perception of it, and using the knowledge and skills available to create, from scratch, a previously untested novel course of action. Creative decision making is not normally something associated with or recommended in high-risk situations (Flin et al, 2008). More creativity in pre-hospital decision making may be required during patient extrication, access and egress to challenging environments or in limb immobilisation techniques, based upon the clinician's individual assessment of the situation.

These four methods of decision making and the benefits and limitations of each are outlined in Table 8.2.

Table 8.2 – Advantages and pitfalls of decision-making methods

	Advantages	Potential Pitfalls
Recognition-primed	<ul><li>Fast</li><li>Requires little effort</li><li>Relatively unaffected by stress</li><li>Reliable in commonly encountered situations</li></ul>	<ul><li>Susceptible to confirmation bias</li><li>Difficult to justify the decision afterwards</li><li>Requires extensive prior experience to be effective</li></ul>
Rule-based	<ul><li>Can be fast, provided that the rule is known</li><li>Useful to inexperienced/novice staff</li><li>Straightforward to explain/justifiable</li><li>Complies with 'best practice'</li></ul>	<ul><li>The 'rule' can be difficult to recall, or find</li><li>Assumes that the 'rule' is up to date</li><li>Only works if the correct 'rule' is chosen</li><li>Possible knowledge or skill decay</li></ul>
Choice	<ul><li>Likely to result in a good choice</li><li>The rationale for the decision can be explained</li><li>Can be supported by decision-making tools</li></ul>	<ul><li>Unhelpful in time-pressured situations</li><li>Cognitively intense</li><li>Challenging when distractions are present</li><li>Can generate 'option paralysis'</li></ul>

(continued)

Table 8.2 – Advantages and pitfalls of decision-making methods (*continued*)

	Advantages	Potential Pitfalls
Creative	<ul><li>Will result in innovative solutions, and possibly new knowledge</li><li>The only option in novel situations</li></ul>	<ul><li>Challenging to justify</li><li>Requires effort</li><li>Requires time</li><li>Very sensitive to distraction</li><li>Possible outcomes are unknown</li><li>Can be difficult to enact if others disagree</li></ul>

Source: Adapted from Flin et al (2008)

Factors that Influence Situation Awareness and Decision Making

In common with other cognitive processes, situation awareness and decision making are inhibited by distractions and interruptions, and can be affected when individuals are hungry, ill, tired, overloaded or stressed. Endsley illustrates a number of factors that influence situation awareness and decision making on her model (Figure 8.12), separating them into individual factors and system factors, but we should accept that these are arbitrary distinctions: the training of an individual, for example, is largely consequent on elements of the system in which that individual trains and practises.

Becoming task fixated (or having tunnel vision) on goals can cause other information not to be perceived. Having a rigid preconception of how a situation will turn out may also have this effect and lead to confirmation bias. Although increased levels of experience and training do not guarantee enhanced situation awareness and decision making, it is likely that experienced practitioners will spend less time and effort formulating mental models, selecting from options, and are able to make more efficient intuitive decisions. Those with less experience may find this more challenging.

An HF/E approach should focus on system design to optimise system factors and support performance. The way in which elements of the work system generate and present the data required for perception and comprehension is relevant. This can be particularly related to technology that ambulance clinicians use to gain information, for example, patient monitors. Stress, fatigue and extremes of workload can decrease capacity to take in new information and affect comprehension and projection, but can be countered by systematic measures such as rota design and rest periods. The complexity of the system in which an individual is trying to make decisions will also have an effect. If the system becomes too complex, it may increase the workload demands to such a level that it exceeds individual capabilities. Automation may reduce the clinician's workload, but technology in the workplace which is designed

Factors that Influence Situation Awareness and Decision Making

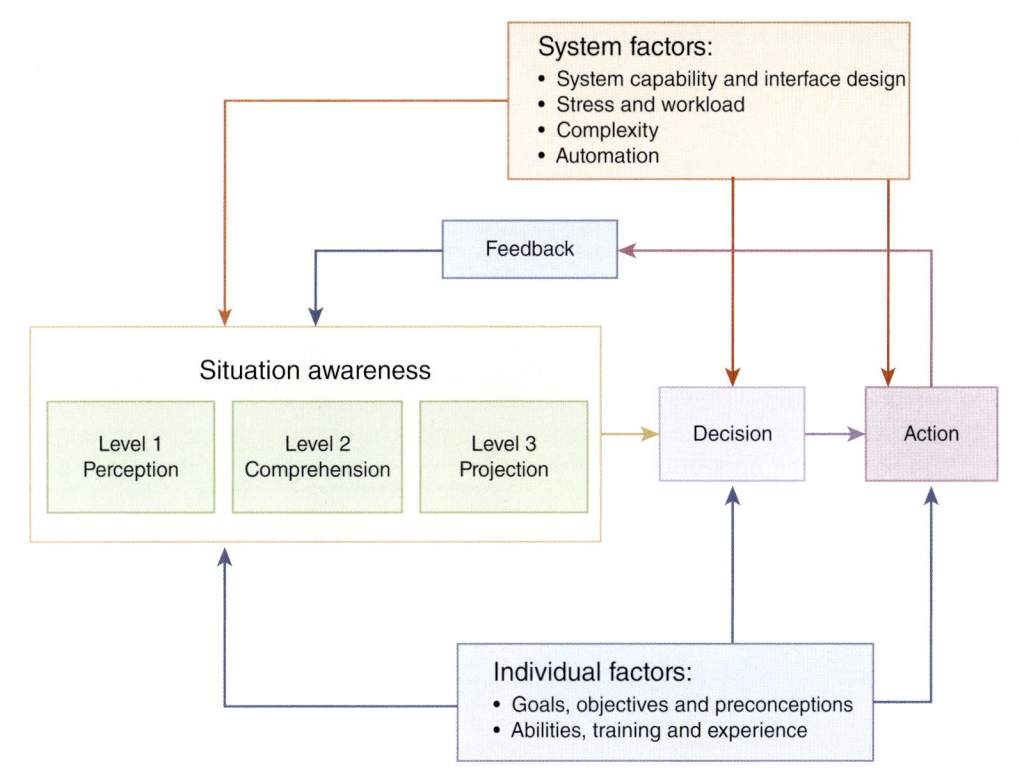

System factors:
- System capability and interface design
- Stress and workload
- Complexity
- Automation

Feedback

Situation awareness
- Level 1 Perception
- Level 2 Comprehension
- Level 3 Projection

Decision → Action

Individual factors:
- Goals, objectives and preconceptions
- Abilities, training and experience

Figure 8.12 – Factors affecting situation awareness
Source: Based on Endsley, 1995

to decrease a person's involvement in the process can instead lead to a decrease in their ability to perceive and respond to changes.

System factors, specifically related to paramedic decision making in 'transition decisions', i.e. decisions that are made in relation to considering triage, referral, non-conveyance and discharge options, have been described by O'Hara et al (2015). They suggest that 'paramedics are reliant on their own professional judgement to interpret ambiguous situations' in relation to non-conveyance decisions, and that there is a need to enhance the understanding of influences on this decision making to ensure safe patient care. Seven ambulance service-specific system influences that affect paramedic decision making in these areas are proposed, with some of these aligning with the factors suggested by Endsley:

- **Increasing demand** – the changing role of ambulance services leads to an increase in non-emergency cases, and subsequently more decisions related to non-conveyance.

- **Inadequate staff training and development** – investment in training and development to support ambulance clinicians in this type of decision making may be lagging behind the pace of change in service demand profiles.

Chapter 8 – Situation Awareness and Decision Making

- **Organisational performance priorities** – UK ambulance services have traditionally measured performance on response time targets, although most services have been introducing a range of clinical performance indicators. It was noted that paramedics were aware of pressures related to measurement of 'on scene' times and non-conveyance rates, although experienced paramedics may be able to resist this influence.

- **Availability and access to alternative care pathways** – in instances where it may be more appropriate not to convey the patient to the emergency department, the suboptimal design of the alternative care options or pathways prevented a referral, and resulted in conveyance to hospital.

- **Risk aversion** – preconceptions associated with a lack of managerial support related to undesired outcomes were identified. This may result in the decision to convey the patient to hospital, rather than explore other options, in order to avoid 'getting it wrong'.

- **Communication and feedback to staff** – some very useful decision support tools and mechanisms exist, for example, for ST elevation myocardial infarctions, trauma and stroke cases. Views on professional-to-professional decision-making support was reported to be mixed, with variable experiences of communication with GPs, out-of-hours services and falls teams. Crucially, it was suggested that a lack of feedback to individual paramedics related to previous non-conveyance decisions was a real barrier to individual and system learning.

- **Resources** – ambulance services require to be suitably resourced with sufficient staff, vehicles and equipment to meet demand and support safe decision making.

Summary

Situation awareness and decision making are cognitive non-technical skills that enhance and complement an ambulance clinician's technical skills. They are closely linked and enable paramedics to take in information from the world around them, make sense of it and decide what, if anything, should happen next. These are small but important elements of the HF/E discipline as they are related to how humans perform and cognitively interact with other elements of the work system, such as colleagues, patients, equipment and the environment. Ideally, where possible, the work environment, technology and processes should be designed to maximise the non-technical skills of those working on the frontline in pre-hospital care.

References

Bennett, R., Mehmed, N., Williams, B. (2020). Non-technical skills in paramedicine: A scoping review. *Nursing and Health Sciences* [online]. Availble from: doi: 10.1111/nhs.12765.

Buchanan, D., Huczynski, A. (2019). *Organizational Behaviour*. 10th Ed. Harlow: Pearson Education.

Civil Aviation Authority (2013). *Global Fatal Accident Review 2002 to 2011: CAP 1036*. West Sussex: The Stationery Office.

Civil Aviation Authority (2016). *Flight-Crew Human Factors Handbook: CAP 737*. West Sussex: CAA.

College of Paramedics (2017). *Paramedic Curriculum Guidance*. 4th Ed. Bridgwater: College of Paramedics.

Collen, A. (2017). *Decision Making in Paramedic Practice*. Bridgwater: Class Professional Publishing.

Croskerry, P., Singahl, G., Mamede, S. (2013). Cognitive debiasing 1: origins of bias and theory of debiasing. *BMJ Quality & Safety*. 22: 58–64.

Dekker, S.W.A. (2015). The danger of losing situation awareness. *Cognitive Technology and Work*. 17(2): 159–161.

Endsley, M.R. (1995). Towards a theory of situation awareness in dynamic systems. *Human Factors*. 37(1): 32–64.

Flin, R., O'Connor, P., Crichton, M. (2008). *Safety at the Sharp End: A guide to non-technical skills*. Aldershot: Ashgate.

Fortune, P.M. et al. (2013). *Human Factors in the Healthcare Setting: A pocket guide for clinical instructors*. West Sussex: Wiley Blackwell.

Golightly, D. (2015). Situation awareness. In: Wilson, J.R., Sharples, S. (eds). *Evaluation of Human Work*. 4th Ed. Boca Raton: CRC Press, pp. 549–563.

Gregory, R.L., Heard, P. (1979). Border locking and the Café Wall illusion. *Perception*. 8(4): 365–380.

Grissinger, M. (2015). Sidetracks on the safety express: interruptions lead to errors and ... wait, what was I doing? *Pharmacy and Therapeutics*. 40(3): 145–190.

Hearns, S. (2019). *Peak Performance Under Pressure*. Bridgwater: Class Professional Publishing.

Hunter, J., Porter, M., Williams, B. (2019). What Is Known About Situational Awareness in Paramedicine? A Scoping Review. *Journal of Allied Health*. 48(1): 27–34.

Hunter, J., Porter, M., Williams, B. (2020). Towards a theoretical framework for situational awareness in paramedicine. *Safety Science*. 122: 104528.

Jégoux, F.-M. (2018). Developing non-technical skills. *HindSight*. 27: 21–23. Brussels: EUROCONTROL.

Jensen, J.L. et al. (2016). A survey to determine decision-making styles of working paramedics and student paramedics. *Canadian Journal of Emergency Medicine*. 18(3): 213–222.

Joint Royal Colleges Ambulance Liaison Committee, Association of Ambulance Chief Executives (2019). *JRCALC Clinical Guidelines 2019*. Bridgwater: Class Professional Publishing.

Kahneman, D. (2012). *Thinking, Fast and Slow*. London: Penguin Books.

Klein, G. (2008). Naturalistic decision making. *Human Factors*. 50(3): 456–460.

Lauria, M.J., Ghobrial, M.K., Hicks, C.M. (2019). Force of habit: developing situation awareness in critical care transport. *Air Medical Journal*. 38: 45–50.

Müller-Lyer, F.C. (1889). Optische Urtheilstäuschungen. *Archiv für Physiologie Suppl*. 263–270.

O'Hara, R. et al. (2015). A qualitative study of systematic influences on paramedic decision making: care transitions and patient safety. *Journal of Health Services Research & Policy*. 20(1): 45–53.

Chapter 8 – Situation Awareness and Decision Making

Perona, M., Rahman, M.A., O'Meara, P. (2019). Paramedic judgement, decision-making and cognitive processing: a review of the literature. *Australasian Journal of Paramedicine*. 16: 1–12 [online]. Available from: https://ajp.paramedics.org/index.php/ajp/article/view/586/783

Resuscitation Council (UK) (2015). Adult advanced life support algorithm [online]. Available from: https://www.resus.org.uk/resuscitation-guidelines/adult-advanced-life-support/#algorithm

Ryan, L., Halliwell, D. (2012). Paramedic decision-making: how is it done? *Journal of Paramedic Practice*. (6): 343–351.

Shields, A., Flin, R. (2013). Paramedics' non-technical skills: a literature review. *Emergency Medicine Journal*. 30(5): 350–354.

Stanton, N.A. et al. (2010). Is situation awareness all in the mind? *Theoretical Issues in Ergonomic Science*. 11(1–2): 29–40.

Stanton, N.A. et al. (2017). State-of-science: situation awareness in individuals, teams and systems. *Ergonomics*. 60(4): 449–466.

Chapter 9
Teamwork in Paramedic Practice
Mike Christian and Neil Jeffers

> In this chapter:
> - Forming teams
> - Shared cognition in teamwork
> - Tools and techniques that can be adopted in pre-hospital teams

Scenario

Olu, a 55-year-old man, is crossing the high street when he is suddenly struck by a white van travelling at 50 mph, throwing him 7 feet into the air before landing in a crumpled pile on the edge of the road 15 feet away. The impact with the vehicle has broken his right femur, smashed his pelvis and fractured multiple ribs on the right side of his chest, two of which have punctured his lung. Upon landing on the road his head has struck the kerb causing impact brain apnoea, resulting in him losing consciousness. Combined with the position of his head, this is obstructing his airway and has left him breathing ineffectively. As the van rushes off, a bystander calls 999.

The police and ambulance dispatchers alert their closest staff: Tom, a police traffic sergeant nearing retirement; Leila, an ambulance officer (paramedic) in a response car with 20 years' experience who recently returned to the 'road' after spending the past five years leading a quality improvement initiative; and Noor (newly qualified paramedic) and Jemma (EMT [Emergency Medical Technician], 15 years' experience) who are partnered today for the first time on an ambulance as Jemma's usual partner is on leave. This team, who have never met before, are required to execute a number of time-critical actions and get Olu to the Emergency Department or he will die. Similar scenarios to that above are played out thousands of times each day around the world both in the pre-hospital environment and during emergencies in hospitals and other industries.

Introduction

Any team performing a task together must address issues encountered at the individual level as well as at the team level. Paramedics and other emergency responders face a particularly unique additional challenge related to the formation

Chapter 9 – Teamwork in Paramedic Practice

of teams. If one was planning to create a high performance team to attempt to save Olu's life you would never design a team by randomly assigning people with no thought to their individual skill sets or team composition, let alone not introduce the team before the event or provide them with an opportunity to train and practise together. Therefore, an HF/E approach to teamwork would be to consider the interactions between team members, how to design the team and the way it trains, to optimise its function for well-being and system performance. However, this can be challenging in pre-hospital care.

Teamwork in emergency domains is recognised as beneficial for patient safety, with several key principles proposed:

- Team leadership is vital.
- Team members must have clear roles and responsibilities.
- Shared understanding and mental models with team-mates are beneficial.
- Pre-briefing and debriefing should be incorporated.
- Team trust and psychological safety should not be underestimated.
- Training in communication techniques increases team performance.
- Achieving a common vision of the team's goals enhances effectiveness.
- Teams that learn from experiences and are adaptable deal better with non-routine, stressful situations.

(Salas et al, 2007)

This chapter will use these principles as a backdrop when discussing team formation, key team non-technical skills and interactions related to team performance, including shared situation awareness and decision making, authority gradients, communication, task management and leadership within teams. In particular, these factors will be considered with the above case study in mind. However, the principles discussed can be applied in many other situations where ambulance clinicians work in teams. Throughout the chapter it is important to remember that having a team is not only important in order to facilitate the number of tasks which must be achieved within a compressed time frame (many hands make light work) but also the team members themselves serve as redundant systems to monitor and back up each other (a safety function) (Wilson et al, 2010).

Forming Teams

Teams are generally defined using phrases that include 'group of people' as well as a 'common goal', 'common task' or 'common good'. Although it is important to have a 'common goal' when forming a team in a crisis, it is essential to recognise from the outset that problems are likely to arise if you naively assume that all responders to the emergency (your 'team') automatically share the same priorities. Each person's version of 'good' (top priority) might be different. From the incident described at the beginning of the chapter, at the outset of the response Tom's top priority may be to

Forming Teams

secure evidence to identify the driver of the white van, while Leila's priority may be to manage the scene (and perhaps avoid direct patient care), whereas Noor's priority may be to avoid making any mistakes given this is one of her first major trauma patients since graduation, and Jemma perhaps has a priority of not appearing to be clinically 'out-dated' compared with her partner today, a new university graduate. Thus, before this group can ever truly become a team they must align on a common top priority: 'to save Olu's life'. To understand the process of team formation a little better let's take a moment to consider how teams form in non-emergency situations and some of the factors that affect that process.

The process of group development in non-emergency situations proposed by Tuckman (1965) (Figure 9.1) remains one of the most widely accepted today. Tuckman points out that small groups may be characterised either by appointed or emergent leadership.

In emergency situations, however, particularly in the pre-hospital environment, most teams don't have the luxury of dedicating very much time to the forming, storming or norming stages as they must rapidly get to the 'performing' stage in order to deliver critical interventions effectively to help patients. Under ideal circumstances a team will be constituted and have an opportunity to go through these stages prior to facing an emergency (Mercer et al, 2014). Nonetheless, this model helps us understand that creating a team to achieve a task is not a simple process, nor one free of potential interpersonal challenges and conflict. Realising this is key to understanding and addressing potential issues within a team. The first step of course is to understand yourself, how you communicate, how you handle conflict, and your leadership and followership styles. Collaboration in the team context has been described as:

> ... learning to identify team members' strengths and weaknesses, understanding individual's personal expectations and the expectations of other team members, then forming a system that supports using the strengths, developing the weaknesses where appropriate, and deciding which personal expectations can be fulfilled while working together successfully.
>
> (Van Stephoudt and Mariotta, 2013)

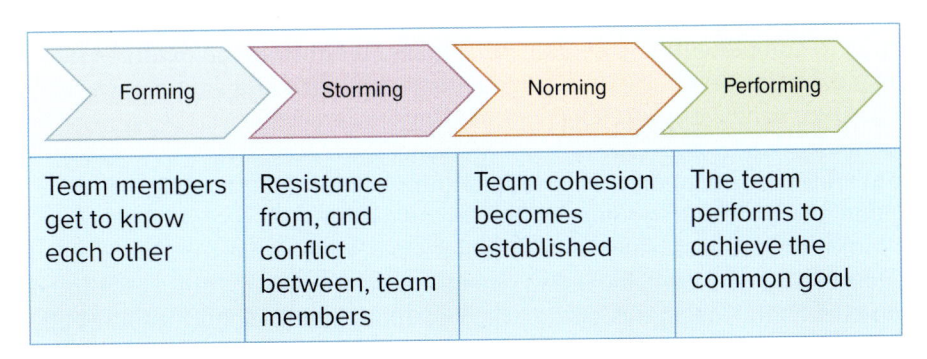

Forming	Storming	Norming	Performing
Team members get to know each other	Resistance from, and conflict between, team members	Team cohesion becomes established	The team performs to achieve the common goal

Figure 9.1 – Team formation stages
Source: Based on Tuckman (1965)

The team formation stage is critical and impacts the care provided to patients. It has been demonstrated that simply staggering the arrival of responders to a simulated cardiac arrest decreases overall team performance, and patient outcome, compared with the responders being together with the patient for even just a few moments before the emergency occurs (Hunziker et al, 2009, 2011). Some factors suggested to have a negative impact on team performance include communication issues, confirmation bias, hierarchy issues and changes in leadership. Unfortunately, limited research is currently available to inform the best way to build an 'ad hoc' team during an emergency, with responders joining the team at staggered intervals. One of the first steps, however, is to recognise that 'jumping right in' when you as a responder arrive on scene with a team that has already partially formed can potentially have negative effects. Often it is useful to at least briefly survey the scene from the periphery and attempt to judge if a critical intervention is in process or not and if the existing team is ready to 'on-board' you, or whether it is better to make your presence known and wait to be invited to the team and tasked with a responsibility. Similarly, if you are of a 'higher status', for instance a more senior clinician or supervisor, and upon your assessment the current leader is performing well, it may lead to better results if you do not take over the leadership but remain in a supportive role posing questions or coaching, rather than assuming control and giving directions (Hunziker, 2011). Ad hoc team formation during emergencies is an area that would benefit greatly from future research.

Team Situation Awareness and Decision Making

Situation awareness and mental models, as described in Chapter 8, are states of perception and understanding held within the mind of an individual. In a team these states must be shared between individuals in order for a team to function effectively. Endsley (2010) describes the need for a team to perceive critical factors in their environment and to comprehend what those factors mean, particularly when integrated together in relation to the team's goals, as well as have an understanding of what will (or is expected to) happen in the near future. It is important to recognise that shared situation awareness and team situation awareness are not simply the summative components of the individual team member's situation awareness (Figure 9.2). If one team member has a more established situation awareness, this does not compensate for another person's incomplete situation awareness. Each team member must have sufficient situation awareness to complete their own individual tasks. Team situation awareness is overarching and is contributed to by each member's individual situation awareness (Endsley, 1995; Schulz et al, 2013).

Similar to individual situation awareness, gathering information, interpreting information and anticipating future states are all actions that are required to achieve team situation awareness. A number of requirements are necessary for these tasks to be successfully achieved, including accessing the necessary data, comprehending this data and, finally, using this data to project future states (Schulz et al, 2013). Figure 9.3 illustrates these team requirements through the three levels of Endsley's model, discussed in Chapter 8.

Team Situation Awareness and Decision Making

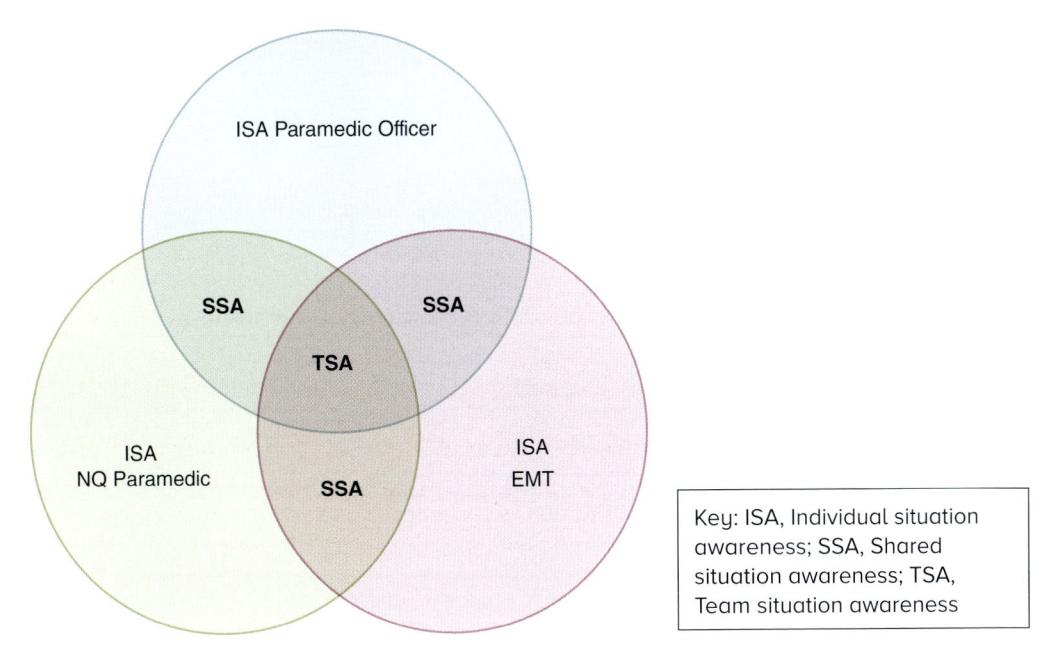

Figure 9.2 – Strata of situation awareness
Source: Based on Endsley (1995) and Schulz et al (2013)

Key: ISA, Individual situation awareness; SSA, Shared situation awareness; TSA, Team situation awareness

Perception
- Other team members, actions and communications
- Shared environment
- Shared technology displays

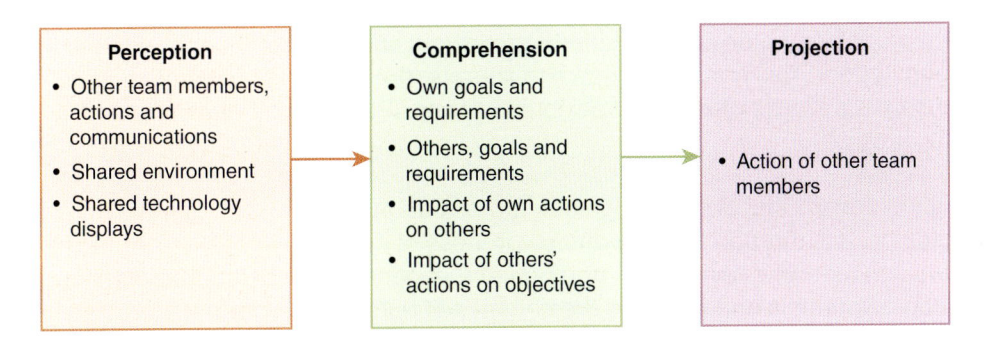

Comprehension
- Own goals and requirements
- Others, goals and requirements
- Impact of own actions on others
- Impact of others' actions on objectives

Projection
- Action of other team members

Figure 9.3 – Team situation awareness requirements
Source: Adapted from Schulz et al (2013)

In attempting to build situation awareness for the team, elements such as communication, shared technology displays and a shared environment can be used. Communication will be further discussed later in this chapter. However, three communication tools which are helpful specifically in building and maintaining team situation awareness are worth mentioning here. These tools are briefs, huddles and situation reports ('sit-reps') (Figure 9.4).

Briefs are used for planning and are typically done when the team first forms. This can of course be a challenge in situations where teams form gradually over time, or when the performance of an urgent clinical intervention is perceived to be a higher

Chapter 9 – Teamwork in Paramedic Practice

Briefs	Huddles	Sit-reps
• Form the team • Designate roles and responsibilities • Establish climate and goals • Short- and long-term planning	• Occur ad hoc • Discuss critical issues • Anticipate outcomes and contingencies • Redistribute resources	• Succinct • Scheduled • Structured

Figure 9.4 – Communication tools for building team situation awareness

priority. Despite this, it is still often useful to hold a brief early in an incident when at least a critical mass of team members is present. Huddles, conversely, are used as required to deal with new information or arising issues. Finally, sit-reps are a tool for sharing information most commonly on a scheduled basis, which may be on a time interval or anchored to a trigger in activities. Sit-reps should be succinct and structured.

A particularly useful concept for facilitating team situation awareness is the notion of a shared mental model for the team. One of the primary benefits of establishing a shared mental model is that it allows members of the team to have a common understanding of the team goals and how they are going to be achieved (the direction of travel). This can enable them to anticipate what tasks are required and to then proactively plan and execute them without specific direction for each task by the team leader. This has been shown to improve the efficiency of communication and the effectiveness of teams in performing tasks (Petrosoniak and Hicks, 2013; Schulz et al, 2013).

As highlighted in Chapter 8, recognition that situation awareness has been lost is challenging. It is through training and awareness of non-technical skills that expert leaders can learn the techniques and gain the experience necessary to monitor situation awareness and increase the chances of recognising when it has been lost. There are several flags described in Chapter 8 that team members, and in particular the team leader, should monitor for, which suggest that individual and/or team situation awareness may be 'lost' or suboptimal. If any of these flags are recognised then it is essential that the team react and work to regain, or rebuild (Figure 9.5) the team situation awareness: this can be accomplished by calling a huddle and reconstructing the shared mental model. It is important that all members of the team

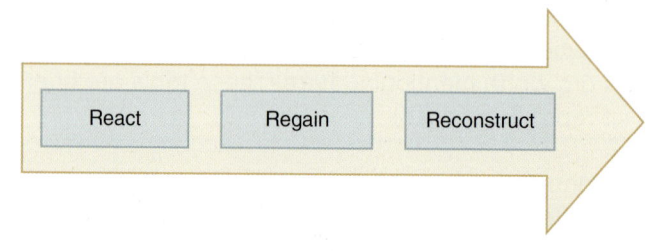

React → Regain → Reconstruct

Figure 9.5 – Response to loss of team situation awareness

feel empowered to declare that team situation awareness has been lost and request for it to be reconstructed. This can be achieved through establishment of a shallow authority gradient (discussed later in the chapter).

However, the timing of this activity is important as it may delay critical tasks, thus it falls to the team leader to consider all aspects and prioritise when it is best to call the huddle. Rather than being in a reactive mode when team situation awareness is lost, it is preferable for the team leader to use tools such as the self-questioning technique suggested in Chapter 8 to optimise individual and team situation awareness.

Despite whether decisions in a situation are being made by an individual or as a collective, the quality of the decisions made are inextricably linked to team situation awareness (Endsley, 1995), and this impacts the decisions both through the accuracy of the information upon which they are based and the context in which they are made. It has been illustrated how inaccurate information derived from the team situation awareness can lead to poor or incorrect decisions being made. The context of the situation, as framed by the team situation awareness, also influences which process of decision making is selected (Endsley, 1995). We know that factors such as urgency (time pressure) of situations have an impact on which of the various methods of decision making are utilised. In low time pressure situations, a slower and more deliberate analytical method of decision making may be used, whereas in high time pressure situations a naturalistic form of decision making, such as recognition-primed decision making, may be employed. These principles also apply to team situation awareness and decision making.

Task Management and Leadership

One of the key roles of leadership in a team is to distribute the workload and harness the individual abilities of the team members to accomplish the objective at hand. These are referred to as task allocation and task management. Task allocation is defined as 'directing specific workers to engage in specific tasks in numbers appropriate to the current situation' (LeSage et al, 2011). Task management denotes a larger process and includes task allocation at its core (illustrated in Figure 9.6) but is more broadly defined as 'managing resources and organising tasks to achieve goals' (Fletcher et al, 2004). While the terms task allocation and task management have different foci, they are often used synonymously. Other terms that can also be commonly used, or overlap in literature, are 'task co-ordination', 'task/workload distribution', 'priority setting' and 'co-ordinating team actions'.

As task allocation is only one step, task management means far more than determining 'who does what'. Whenever there are multiple steps, there is an increased chance of things going wrong, and greater co-ordination is required for things to go right (Scerri et al, 2005; Castelao et al, 2015). A leader can be able and quick at task allocation but still perform suboptimal overall task management. This might be because they did not prioritise the correct first task (due to insufficient situation awareness), did not assign a backup strategy (due to insufficient preparation) or did not confirm that tasks were completed (due to insufficient communication).

Chapter 9 – Teamwork in Paramedic Practice

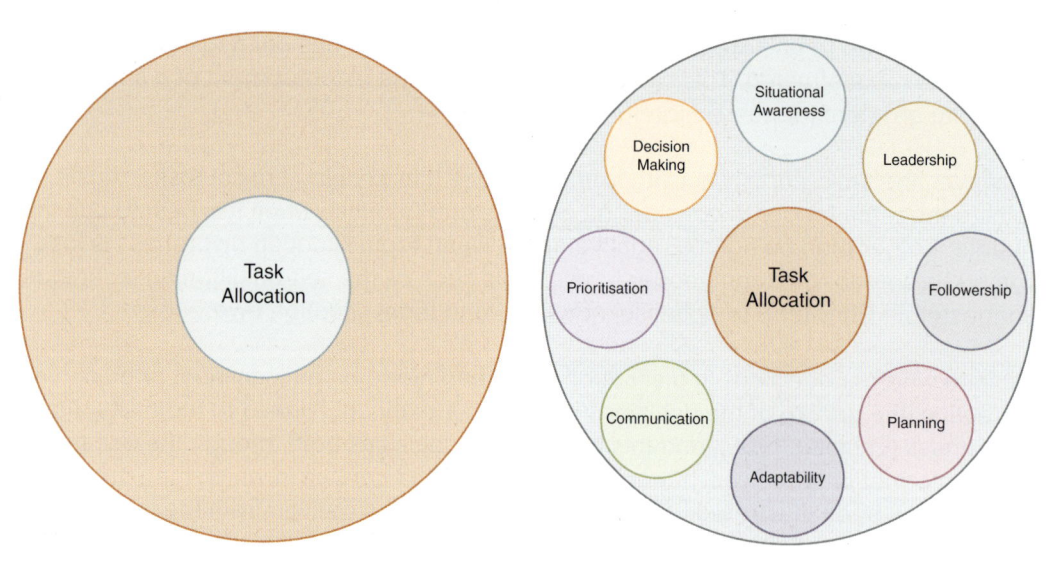

Figure 9.6 – Task allocation vs Task management

Failures in task management can have significant consequences for team performance and have even been linked to deaths of patients as well as emergency responders (Hicks et al, 2008; LeSage et al, 2011). To fully understand the factors that influence task management it is helpful to briefly discuss the cognitive task load (CTL) model (Figure 9.7) proposed by Grootjen et al (2006).

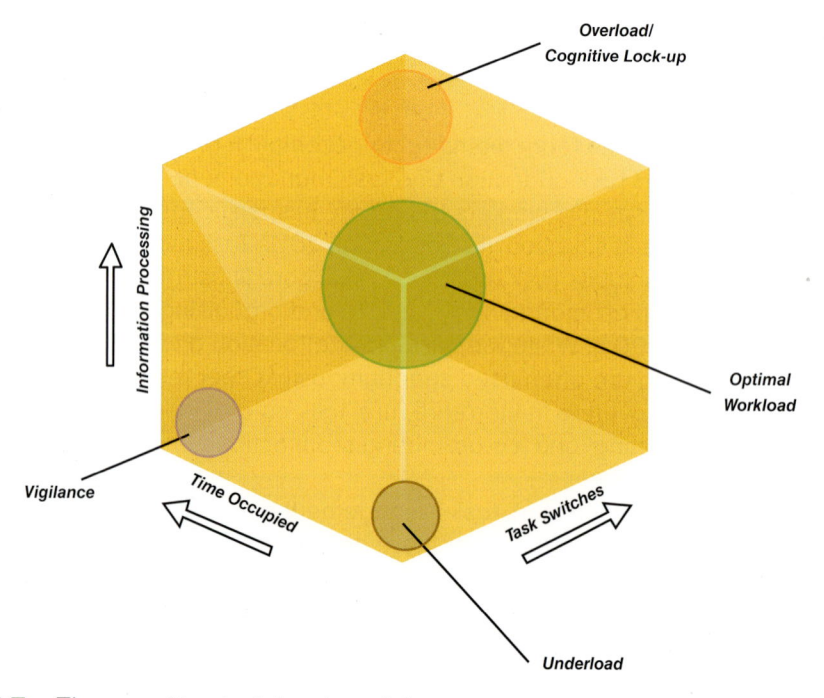

Figure 9.7 – The cognitive task load model
Source: Based on Grootjen et al (2006)

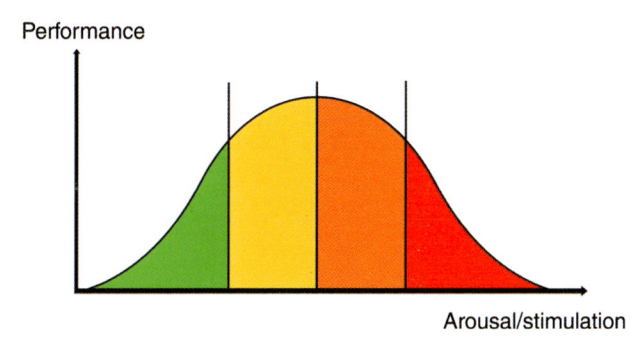

Figure 9.8 – Yerkes–Dodson model
Source: Based on Staal (2004)

The CTL model suggests that people undertaking a performance task will exist in one of four states: optimal workload, underload, overload or vigilance. Optimal workload is when you are 'in the zone', sometimes referred to as 'flow' in psychology, where a state of peak arousal and performance is achieved (Hearns, 2019). The other three states are all less than optimal and include 'overload' where you might see people freeze up, 'underload' where people are essentially bored due to understimulation, and 'vigilance' where you are like a coiled spring ready to launch into action but not actually delivering any output. These states described by the CTL model align closely with the 'bandwidth' concepts described by the Yerkes–Dodson law (Staal, 2004) (Figure 9.8). Bandwidth is a computer analogy that attempts to explain the amount of 'brain power' that could be devoted to tasks and the detriment of being overloaded. Loosely based on the work of Yerkes and Dodson, this concept explains the difference between subjects who are under- or overaroused/stimulated and their response to this. Being in a low bandwidth state, at first glance, seems to be a good place to be with bandwidth spare to devote to other tasks. Clearly being overloaded in a high bandwidth state is bad as the paramedic could suffer from various effects, including 'target fixation' and 'action slip' (discussed later in the chapter). Bandwidth usage can sometimes be referred to in terms of the percentage that is being devoted to the tasks. Let us consider conceptual percentages of 30%, 80% and 100% bandwidth usage.

Thirty percent bandwidth describes a time of low arousal/stimulation, which can actually be suboptimal. As humans we rely on previous observations, memories and mental models to interpret new experiences. In low bandwidth state we suffer from reduced scanning and pattern recognition and therefore we are less able to identify and react to new events. Eighty percent bandwidth is proposed to be the optimum state for effective operation in all environments and it describes the person as optimally aroused/stimulated with a small amount of bandwidth to devote to subtle changes. Eventually the subject reaches 100% bandwidth. Clearly any further stimulation or requirement for extra cognition would overload the person. The first symptom of reaching 100% bandwidth is the loss of listening, as opposed to loss of hearing. The person would be observed by others to be 'in a world of their own' and not capable of listening to what is being said. This may lead to a loss of situation

Chapter 9 – Teamwork in Paramedic Practice

awareness. Other symptoms of reaching 100% bandwidth include target fixation, action slip and environmental capture.

Target fixation: This describes the inability of the person to draw their attention from a specific element of the task, to the detriment of everything else. Quite often this is an easy win or a problem that has been solved before. Tracking down the many variables that render the oxygen saturation probe ineffective is an example.

Action slip: Action slips are unintentional behaviours that are a result of failure to 'pay attention' due to a high bandwidth state. Refer back to Chapter 3 for slip, trip and lapse types of 'errors'.

Environmental capture: This is the situation whereby an action is carried out within the correct environment, however, the action was not the intended one. This has been observed many times when a pilot has incorrectly operated the gear lever, raising the gear instead of lowering it.

In addition to the issues discussed above, three further factors that affect task performance, and therefore have implications for the overall team's performance include:

- the amount of time a person is occupied on a task
- how often a person is required to switch between different tasks
- the amount of bandwidth 'information processing' needed to complete the task.

(Grootjen et al, 2006)

Several factors can have an impact on the leader's ability to manage the tasks which he or she is asking the team to execute. This may include how stable the tasks are, the resources available within the team, the function of team members and the relationships between the tasks (Scerri et al, 2005). Each of these issues are described in more detail below.

Task instability refers to the changing requirement for a task, for example, the need for chest compressions when a patient's condition fluctuates between cardiac arrest and return of spontaneous circulation (ROSC).

Resource limitations must be considered if a single piece of equipment is required for two simultaneous tasks, for example, an ultrasound device for assistance with finding a vein for peripheral IV insertion as well as assessing for a pneumothorax. Requesting two people to do these tasks at the same time with only one ultrasound device available is clearly inefficient task management.

Overlapping functionality refers to the situation where two team members can perform a skill even though they have different overall skill sets which might need to be employed differently. For example, if a paramedic and an EMT (without vascular access insertion skills) are working together to manage a patient who requires both basic airway management (with a BVM and OPA) as well as vascular access, either the paramedic or EMT could perform the basic airway management but only the paramedic could insert the cannula or intra-osseous needle. If the paramedic is initially assigned to do the basic airway management, there will subsequently need to be a change in task roles to gain the vascular access. Thus, it is important for the team leader to assign the tasks appropriately to optimise the overall management of the patient.

Finally, **inter-task constraints** refer to one task (such as gaining IV access) which must be carried out prior to another (such as giving an IV drug). Again, the order of allocation of those tasks is critical for effective task management.

Authority Gradients

An authority gradient, sometimes also called 'command gradient', is an actual or perceived difference in the hierarchy of authority, rank or grade between team members, which can have positive or negative effects. As the senior clinician on scene you might be expected to lead, sometimes follow and occasionally just do as instructed. Understanding and appreciating the advantages and limitations related to the steepness of the authority gradient is key to utilising the concept for the benefit of teamwork. If the gradient is too steep it could inhibit communication, undermine the shared mental model and could lead to adverse consequences. Conversely, an appropriately steep authority gradient can be a good thing, as sometimes team members will benefit from direct and positive instruction.

Steep authority gradients were evident in a number of significant aviation incidents in the late 1970s. In 1978 a plane took off from New York JFK and flew to Portland, Oregon. The weather was good. As they approached their destination and tried to put down the undercarriage, they encountered a problem. The crew was comprised of an experienced captain, a co-pilot and a flight engineer. Among them they had more than enough skills, knowledge and time (given the fuel status) to solve this problem. However, the crew worked to resolve the undercarriage problem for over an hour, reducing fuel levels to dangerously low levels. Although the fuel situation was noticed by the co-pilot and flight engineer, neither of them were able to change the course of action given the perceived authority gradient between them and the captain. The plane ran out of fuel, all four engines stopped and the plane crashed killing 10 people and injuring 74 (National Transport Safety Board, 1979). This type of situation unfortunately is not unique to aviation and is a common factor identified in healthcare safety incidents. Michaels et al (2007) explain that, in most surgical adverse events, someone knew that something was wrong but either did not speak up or was ignored. It would be easy to imagine that authority gradients can be a factor in pre-hospital settings due to either 'clinical grade' (students, emergency ambulance crew, technician, paramedic, doctor, and so on) or due to 'administrative rank' (ambulance officers). This gradient in teams can be mitigated through selection, training and use of communication tools. Ideally, leaders who can demonstrate skills in establishing appropriate authority gradients should be selected, and teams should

Chapter 9 – Teamwork in Paramedic Practice

train together to understand optimal gradients for different situations. Team leaders should aim to be receptive to the input and suggestions of others and team members should be appropriately assertive for the situation. Therefore, it is important to arm people with the tools to overcome the problems of a steep authority gradient when it does occur. Some simple communication tools to address this will be covered in the final section of this chapter.

Communication

Communication is a group (team) activity as it requires two or more parties to be involved. Given that communication is a skill most of us practise on a daily basis, we often take for granted the complexity of the act of communication to another person (Figure 9.9).

Failure can occur at each step in the communication process, commonly resulting in team dysfunction or a failure to achieve the team's goals. Although communication can occur via many different mediums, we will focus on verbal communication within this chapter since it is the most commonly used method in the context of teamwork in paramedic practice. However, it is important to be mindful that communication itself is comprised of more than simply the spoken word. All verbal communication that occurs face-to-face also has a non-verbal component (body language) as well as the tone or sound of the voice. In some circumstances the non-verbal and tone components are responsible for conveying the majority of the message that

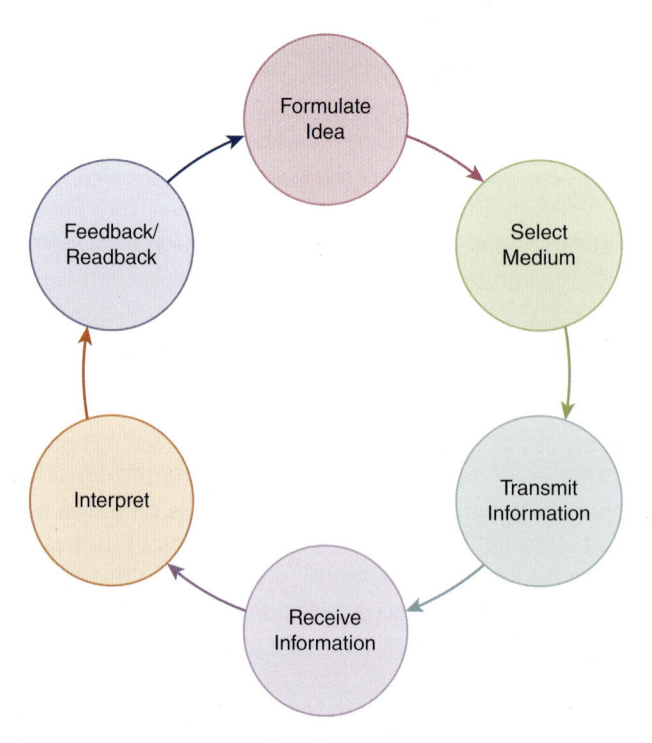

Figure 9.9 – Closed loop communication process

Table 9.1 – Responsibilities in communication

Sender's Responsibilities	Receiver's Responsibilities
• communicate information: Clearly, Correctly, Completely (3Cs) • communicate in a timely manner • request verification or feedback.	• acknowledge communication • repeat information • provide feedback.

is received by the other party involved. For communication to be effective, both parties involved must be accountable for their own responsibilities in the exchange (Table 9.1). Communication is a tool to be used to achieve a number of important functions within the team context (Kanki, 2010).

In an effort to improve team communication, the 'SBAR' tool (originally designed for use in the US military to call in air support) has become widely adopted within healthcare as a useful tool to pass on information (Leonard et al, 2004). Sometimes a second 'R' for 'readback' is added. 'SBARR' can be used in a variety of situations when effective communication is of utmost importance, and is best used as a proactive tool to prevent communication failures rather than reserving it for when something has gone wrong. SBARR stands for:

Situation: The problem
- What is going on with the patient?

Background: Brief, related, to the point
- What is the clinical background or context?

Assessment: What you found and what you think
- What do I think the problem is?

Recommendation: What you want
- What do you need to do your job effectively and safely?

Readback: Receiver acknowledges info given
- Is the summary of the issues/plan consistent with the points above?

As discussed earlier in the chapter, one of the major impediments to effective communication in teams can be the perception of a steep authority gradient. A number of tools have also been developed to overcome situations when a steep authority gradient is potentially impacting team performance. The first tool, referred to as the 'two-challenge rule', was originally developed for the aviation industry but has now gained greater uptake within healthcare. This tool places an onus on the person who has recognised a safety issue to raise it at least twice with the team leader, and if appropriate action does not occur, the team member raising the

Chapter 9 – Teamwork in Paramedic Practice

concern is encouraged to take further action to resolve the situation. In the context of aviation this may mean taking control of the aircraft and undertaking an evasive manoeuvre, or in the healthcare setting this typically means escalating the issue to a higher authority. The 'CUS' tool is also often used in conjunction with the two-challenge rule and is a form of escalating language (Leonard et al, 2004). 'CUS' stands for:

> I'm **C**oncerned
>
> I'm **U**ncomfortable
>
> This is un**S**afe, or I'm **S**cared or **S**top.

An alternative graded assertiveness tool that can be utilised is the 'PACE' tool, which stands for:

> **P**robe: for example, 'Is this right?'
>
> **A**lert: 'I am not sure that this is right'
>
> **C**hallenge: 'This is not right because...'
>
> **E**mergency: 'Stop!' or 'I have control'.

In order for these tools to be most effective, teams must be familiar with their concepts and trained in their use. Again, this presents a challenge in the pre-hospital setting with random team formation but highlights the importance of including basic non-technical skills training in core training for all emergency responders.

Summary

This chapter provides insight into some of the key principles in the way that individuals interact within teams in the pre-hospital work system. Both leaders and team members are critical to enabling the objectives of the team to be achieved. By understanding how teams are formed and being familiar with the concepts of team situation awareness, task allocation, task management and authority gradients, system performance can be enhanced, enabling team members to be more effective in delivering care to patients.

The use and implementation of the various communication tools that have been discussed will be invaluable to addressing challenges that arise in team function and performance. Of greatest importance is the realisation that it is possible to study and learn about these topics as well as to develop and master team skills through training and practise. Therefore, teamwork and other non-technical skills practise and training interventions should be designed with an understanding of the relevant system element interactions. Paramedics should no more accept failures in providing care as a result of people being 'maxed out' or due to 'poor CRM' than they would accept a patient dying with ventricular fibrillation because their defibrillator didn't work. Teams are a tool that can be employed to save lives – like any tool, everyone can develop the skills necessary to use them most effectively.

References

Castelao, E.F. et al. (2015). Effect of CRM team leader training on team performance and leadership behavior in simulated cardiac arrest scenarios: a prospective, randomized, controlled study. *BMC Medical Education.* 15: 116.

Endsley, M.R. (1995). Toward a theory of situation awareness dynamic systems. *Human Factors.* 37(1): 32–64.

Endsley, M.R. (2010). Situation awareness in aviation systems. In: Wise, J., Hopkin, V., Garland, D. (eds). *Handbook of Aviation Human Factors.* 2nd Ed. Boca Raton: CRC Press.

Fletcher, G. et al. (2004). Rating non-technical skills: developing a behavioural marker system for use in anaesthesia. *Cognition, Technology & Work.* 6(3): 165–171.

Grootjen, M., Neerincx, M., Veltman, J.A. (2006). Cognitive task load in a naval ship control centre: From identification to prediction. *Ergonomics.* 49(12–13): 1238–1264.

Hearns, S. (2019). *Peak Performance Under Pressure.* Bridgwater: Class Professional Publishing.

Hicks, C.M., Bandiera, G.W., Denny, C.J. (2008). Building a simulation-based crisis resource management course for emergency medicine, phase 1: Results from an interdisciplinary needs assessment survey. *Academic Emergency Medicine.* 15(11): 1136–1143.

Hunziker, S. et al. (2009). Hands-on time during cardiopulmonary resuscitation is affected by the process of teambuilding: a prospective randomised simulator-based trial. *BMC Emergency Medicine.* 9(3).

Hunziker, S. et al. (2011). Teamwork and leadership in cardiopulmonary resuscitation. *Journal of the American College of Cardiology.* 57(24): 2381–2388.

Kanki, B.G. (2010). Communication and crew resource management. In: Wiener, E.L., Kanki, B.G., Helmreich, R.L. (eds). *Crew Resource Management.* 2nd Ed. San Diego: Academic Press.

Leonard, M., Graham, S., Bonacum, D. (2004). The human factor: the critical importance of effective teamwork and communication in providing safe care. *Quality & Safety in Health Care.* 13(Suppl 1): i85–i90.

LeSage, P., Dyar, J.T., Evans, B.E. (2011). *Crew Resource Management: Principles and Practice.* Sudbury: Jones and Bartlett.

Mercer, S.J., Arul, G., Pugh, H. (2014). Performance improvement through best practice team management: human factors in complex trauma. *Journal of the Royal Army Medical Corps.* 160(2): 105–108.

Michaels, R.K. et al. (2007). Achieving the National Quality Forum's 'Never Events': prevention of wrong site, wrong procedure, and wrong patient operations. *Annals of Surgery.* 245(4): 526–532.

National Transport Safety Board (1979). Aircraft Accident Report NTSB-AAR-79-7 [online]. Available from: https://www.ntsb.gov/investigations/AccidentReports/Reports/AAR7907.pdf

Petrosoniak, A., Hicks, C.M. (2013). Beyond crisis resource management: new frontiers in human factors training for acute care medicine. *Current Opinion in Anaesthesiology.* 26(6): 699–706.

Salas, E., Rosen, M., King, H. (2007). Managing teams managing crises: principles of teamwork to improve patient safety in the emergency room and beyond. *Theoretical Issues in Ergonomics Science.* 8(5): 381–394.

Scerri, P. et al. (2005). Allocating Tasks in Extreme Teams. Conference Paper: 4th International Joint Conference on Autonomous Agents and Multiagent Systems. July 25–29, Utrecht, The Netherlands.

Schulz, C.M. et al. (2013). Situation awareness in anesthesia: concept and research. *Anesthesiology.* 118(3): 729–742.

Chapter 9 – Teamwork in Paramedic Practice

Staal, M.A. (2004). Stress, cognition, and human performance: a literature review and conceptual framework. National Aeronautics amd Space Administration [online]. Available from: https://ntrs.nasa.gov/archive/nasa/casi.ntrs.nasa.gov/20060017835.pdf

Tuckman, B.W. (1965). Developmental sequence in small groups. *Psychological Bulletin*. 63: 384–399.

Van Stephoudt, B., Mariotta, A.B. (2013). Team Manual [online]. Cambridge, MA: Massachusetts Institute of Technology. Available from: http://web.mit.edu/collaborationtbox/manual/Team%20Manual%202013.pdf

Wilson, K.A. et al. (2010). Team process. In: Wise, J., Hopkin, V., Garland, D. (eds). *Handbook of Aviation Human Factors*. 2nd Ed. Boca Raton: CRC Press.

Chapter 10
Learning from Events

Paul Bowie and Gary Rutherford

> In this chapter:
> - Guiding principles that underpin how to learn from complex events using systems thinking
> - The importance of this activity to organisational learning and patient safety
> - The challenge to ambulance services to embed this type of approach as routine practice

Introduction

Learning from events is well-established as a routine safety improvement intervention in many care professions and organisations worldwide, particularly so in secondary care settings (Anderson and Kodate, 2015). Opportunities for organisations to learn from events are many and varied. For example, they can take the form of complaints from patients and families, feedback from staff on everyday work hassles and irritations, reporting of patient safety incidents (i.e. where someone was unintentionally harmed or could have been harmed – a near miss), and proactive surveillance of specific incident occurrence such as so-called 'never events'.

Typically, most of this learning will take place after something has gone wrong, is reported and a subsequent investigation of the event is instigated (McKay et al, 2009). This can be either at the organisational or care team-based levels, where those involved in the event and/or those in a position to influence change seek to understand how and why it happened. Team-based review meetings (sometimes called morbidity and mortality meetings in hospital settings) involve team members coming together to identify improvements that can be implemented to minimise the risk of a future event re-occurrence. Unfortunately, team-based safety meetings and reviews involving frontline ambulance clinicians and control centre staff do not appear to be routinely held in ambulance services in comparison with other out-of-hospital professional care groups, such as general medical practice, community pharmacy and primary care dentistry. This may be due to the challenges of arranging

Chapter 10 – Learning from Events

such meetings for a workforce that is distributed across geographical areas, shift pattern working, demands on the service and a lack of appreciation of the benefits of a team-based approach. This means that the established review processes in ambulance services may continue, i.e. one or two people carry out an investigation by interviewing those involved individually and reviewing sequences of events in isolation, then making recommendations. Therefore, there is arguably a gap in reflective learning practice that could be closed in future to align ambulance service staff with other domains of healthcare. For these other healthcare professions, taking part in constructive team learning when things go wrong provides a forum for meaningful reflection, discussion, analysis and improvement in what should be a non-threatening and empathic environment (Pringle et al, 1995). If done well, it can enhance team working, morale, understanding and communication, all of which helps to build a more positive safety culture (Bowie et al, 2005).

However, event analysis is still a highly important organisational learning activity for ambulance and paramedic services worldwide (Fisher et al, 2015). Regardless of whether this learning takes place at the team or organisational level, there are a range of principles and structured analytical frameworks, based on HF/E, safety science and systems thinking concepts, that are useful prompts for those paramedics and ambulance service staff with management and leadership roles in this area.

In this chapter, we outline a series of guiding principles for ambulance service staff, related to reporting, reviewing and learning from events. While they may usefully benefit frontline professionals, they are primarily aimed at ambulance service managers, educators and others involved in leading or teaching 'patient safety' and overlapping topics (for example, incident analysis, quality improvement or professionalism), as well as leaders involved in devising, drafting and implementing up-to-date safety and risk-related organisational policies. The intention is to offer a range of principles and ideas for 'good practice', rather than a prescriptive methodology of 'how to carry out a review'. Optimal application of these principles would be within the team-based safety meeting approach discussed, although could also be incorporated in more traditional investigations.

Reporting of Events

Develop a Shared Understanding and Interpretation of Terminology

Safety and risk-related terminology are often applied randomly and interchangeably in healthcare, leading to confusion and misunderstanding (Drupsteen et al, 2013). The term 'event' is used in this chapter for convenience and could mean any variant of the following: 'patient safety incident', 'critical incident', 'adverse event', 'near miss', 'never event', 'clinical error', 'serious incident', 'complaint', 'good outcome', 'excellence' and so on. Hence 'event' will purposely remain undefined so that it is left open to develop a shared understanding and interpretation locally, both in terms of its potentially positive and negative connotations, as well as to inform which events are judged to be meaningful and therefore worth reporting and learning about.

Incident Reporting and Learning Systems

Unfortunately, it is evident from research activity that incident reporting and learning systems are probably the most visible and studied safety intervention in healthcare, but with the least empirical evidence of learning and improvement effectiveness (Shojania, 2008). The main goals of healthcare incident reporting systems are laudable and unarguable, i.e. to uncover priority system issues that pose a risk to the organisation and undertake a focused investigation to better inform learning and improvement to minimise, or even eliminate, identified risks. However, the achievement of these goals is routinely beset with significant and often insurmountable problems which add to their complexity.

For Macrae (2016), many of these issues are directly traceable to:

> ... what was lost in translation when incident reporting was adapted from aviation and other safety-critical industries, with fundamental aspects of successful incident reporting systems misunderstood, misapplied or entirely missed in healthcare ... [leaving us] ...with confused and contradictory approaches to reporting and learning, seriously limiting the impact of this potentially powerful safety improvement strategy.

A range of long-standing, frustrating issues that afflict most incident reporting and learning systems have been proposed (Shojania, 2008), but which ultimately need to be addressed by organisational leaders if this intervention is to play the key patient safety role that is intended. These are:

- poor engagement among specific clinical groups such as medical practitioners
- inadequate design and usability of IT systems
- lack of a systems approach to data collection, analyses and learning
- lack of feedback to users
- low detection of priority issues
- reporting of mundane events
- limited user confidence in utility of reporting systems
- time taken to report issues.

From the HF/E perspective, we also need to embed systems thinking in how we design and operate our incident reporting and learning systems so that they are practical and usable for end-users, and produce quality data to enable meaningful organisational learning and care improvements. Ambulance services should be particularly mindful of how to design access to these systems to encourage and enable reporting from a largely mobile and remote workforce, i.e. is it possible for staff to report events from the ambulance without returning to station?

Chapter 10 – Learning from Events

Goode et al (2018) outline four core principles of systems thinking in the design of reporting and learning systems:

- *Principle 1: 'Look up and out' rather than 'down and in'* by collecting data on contributory factors from across and beyond the immediate work system up to and including regulators and government.

- *Principle 2: Identify interactions and relationships* by encouraging end-users to provide data regarding potential interactions between contributory factors both within, and across, system levels. Frequently, it is noticeable that system-wide contributory factor data is collected without attempting to examine and prioritise the interactions between them that give rise to why things went wrong.

- *Principle 3: Avoid focusing exclusively on failures* by enabling end-users to describe how the normal conditions of work contributed to incidents as well as identifying perceived problems, or gaps in defences.

- *Principle 4: Apply a systems lens* by including a methodological framework to report, analyse and represent incidents from a systems thinking perspective.

In the safety leadership of ambulance organisations there needs to be a sense of realism about the benefits, limitations and purpose of reporting systems. A strong awareness of the evidence base outlining the barriers to learning and improvement is crucial (Macrae, 2016) and this knowledge can be applied locally to sense-check the overall utility of your organisational incident reporting system and so direct any necessary improvements. It would be essential to enhance the usability of reporting systems, give timely feedback to reporters and directly and explicitly align incident reporting data with genuine and visible improvements, otherwise staff will become disinterested and sceptical about their value.

Consider Emotional Impacts

The emotional well-being of ambulance clinicians and staff involved in safety incidents may suffer to some extent, and perhaps considerably so in a few cases, given the concept of clinicians as so-called 'second victims' when such events occur. While there may be some debate regarding the appropriateness of using the term 'second victim' for healthcare professionals (Ozeke et al, 2019), it is acknowledged that multiple emotional impacts may be experienced such as guilt, anxiety, depression, increased stress levels, fear of punitive action and professional embarrassment (Wu and Steckelberg, 2012; Dekker, 2013). This could result in the reluctance of staff to highlight relevant events, and may lead to them being highly selective in which ones they report (Bowie et al, 2005), i.e. favouring those perceived to be less sensitive or controversial. Additionally, there may be a lack of willingness, readiness or ability to fully engage in the learning process when events are discussed because of a perceived blame culture. It is therefore important to raise awareness of these potential emotional barriers, in order to support colleagues and build psychological safety (Edmondson et al, 2016), which will contribute to a more effective learning culture.

Reviewing Events

1st and 2nd Stories

The differences between '1st stories' and '2nd stories' (introduced in Chapter 4) in relation to the review and explanations of adverse events are discussed by Cook et al (1998). 1st stories normally emerge quickly after the incident and tend to focus on the individuals who were closest to the final outcome. Shorrock (2017) supports this by stating that 1st stories:

- are focused on a short time period
- adopt a very personalised view which is interested in the individuals
- can fail to consider context and complexity
- can often be the final review of an incident.

The occurrence of an adverse event can understandably cause anxiety for those involved, and for those who have managerial or leadership responsibility for the area or department in which it occurred. These anxieties can often lead to an eagerness to 'fix' the problem and provide reassurance that it won't happen again. Therefore, the quickly appearing 1st story that seems to identify the problem and offer a simple solution can often be embraced, as it will subconsciously alleviate these anxieties.

If reviews and learning stop at this point, there may be a missed opportunity to consider the deeper and wider aspects that the 2nd story reveals. Where the 1st story offers a quick and simple problem identification and solution, the 2nd story:

- emerges slowly after the event
- focuses on a longer time period
- is less concerned with individual actions
- is more interested in interactions between elements of the complex system, and system vulnerability.

The 2nd story is one that can be uncovered when investigators pursue it, and it can lead to more effective learning and systems improvement (Cook et al, 1998). Interestingly, a 2nd story is often less newsworthy and rarely attracts the same level of media interest as a 1st story would (Shorrock, 2017). Therefore, when an incident occurs in pre-hospital care and a review is commissioned, more organisational learning will take place if the investigator or review team are aware of the profile that the 1st story will likely receive, but anticipate its limitations and explore further to understand the 2nd story.

Avoid Blaming Others (and Yourself) to Move Beyond 'Human Error' as a 'Root Cause'

Blaming colleagues (directly or indirectly), or even yourself, when something goes wrong is frequently misplaced and is counterproductive to learning, improving

Chapter 10 – Learning from Events

safety and developing and sustaining cordial relationships in the workplace (McNab et al, 2016). Our instinctive urge to blame in these circumstances is for many a natural human reaction. Indeed, a proportion of clinicians tend to view the 'causes' of incidents as being mainly attributable to their own actions or inactions, which is contrary to modern safety science theory. But as part of our approach to our professionalism in the workplace we need to self-check and manage our intuitive reactions at these times, and to remember the general axiom that we and our colleagues do not purposefully go to work 'to do a bad job' (Dekker, 2006).

As discussed in Chapter 3, the problem of 'human error' (or 'paramedic error') is viewed largely as a misnomer in HF/E science because it is highly likely to be a symptom of a problem in the wider care system. From this perspective, 'human error' is not the 'cause' of the event and arguably we should avoid using the term in this context (despite its widespread use by the media, judiciary and others). If you arrive at a judgement of 'human error' then it needs to be recognised that this is the starting point for learning from the related event and not its conclusion.

Integrate 'Systems Thinking' in the Analytical Process

As discussed in Chapter 4, most healthcare settings, including pre-hospital care, are viewed as a complex socio-technical system – that is, clinical performance and the delivery of care services can only be achieved through the interactions between technical, human, social and organisational components of the system, and these interactions are rarely simple or linear. Examples of common 'complex' attributes of this type of socio-technical system that will resonate with paramedics may include:

- clinical decisions often being made with imprecise information
- individual and team actions varying dependent on conditions to ensure successful and safe outcomes
- system conditions being dynamic, sometimes chaotic and changing rapidly – they cannot always be predicted
- patient demand increasing or changing; for instance, winter pressures, spikes in emergency calls, pandemics or changes in other healthcare systems
- workforce capacity changing, for example, as a result of staff absence or resource cuts
- the wishes and health of patients changing, thereby influencing our understanding and clinical management.

Thinking across the system about these types of interactions, adaptations and levels of complexity is fundamental to the systems-centred approach to learning from events (Goode et al, 2018). The event analysis process itself ultimately directs the depth of understanding as to how and why the event occurred, as well as the identification of learning needs and potential risk management solutions. Rather than simply 'brainstorming' reasons for the event and possible solutions as a group, you should consider applying a systems-based guiding framework that is accessible for

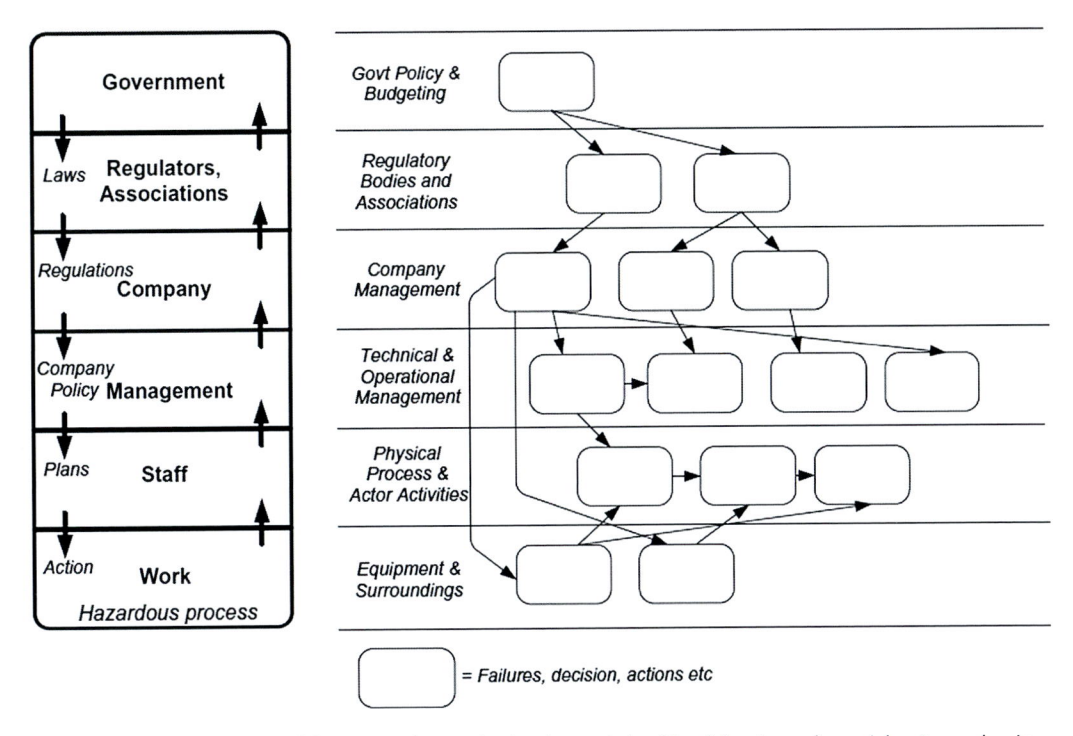

Figure 10.1 – The AcciMaps socio-technical model of incident and accident analysis
Source: Rasmussen (1997); Rasmussen and Svedung, (2000). From Hulme et al, 2019, reproduced with permission.

reviewers (for example, AcciMaps, SEIPS, STEW), although additional training may be required.

The SEIPS and STEW models were discussed in Chapter 4 as tools to help understand system interaction and everyday function when things are going well, or not. AcciMaps (Figure 10.1) is an approach that has been used across a range of industries to specifically understand the role of complex interactions at all system levels in contributing to why things go wrong. This approach contrasts with linear cause and effect models that can often be used when reviewing adverse events in healthcare (for example, root cause analysis tools such as Fishbone diagrams or the 'Five Whys'). Socio-technical models of incident analysis appear to be rarely applied in healthcare, and using other methods means that issues can be overlooked. A systems thinking approach using these tools (SEIPS, STEW, AcciMaps) would encourage us to:

Recognise that Outcomes are 'Emergent'

In the vast majority of cases, it is the complex and dynamic interactions between different system elements that invariably contribute to why things go wrong (and right), rather than the sole actions or inactions of a single individual, regardless of whether this person is 'implicated' in the event in some way, i.e. simply because they were the last person to consult with or treat the patient (Dekker, 2006; Braithwaite et

Chapter 10 – Learning from Events

al, 2015). Events and outcomes from these complex system interactions are therefore said to be 'emergent' rather than caused by a failure of a specific element. 'Emergent' does not mean that something happens by 'magic', but rather in a way that cannot be explained by linear, decomposition and causality principles (Hollnagel et al, 2015).

Explore Situational and Contextual Issues

Generally speaking, situational factors are largely 'factual' and are connected to the circumstances of the incident (before, during and after) in terms of location, space and time. Examples that may be worth exploring include:

- the time of the incident
- levels of workload and patient demand
- staffing levels/mix
- leadership and supervision issues
- the complexity and fitness for purpose of the work tasks
- the availability and functioning of equipment
- adequacy of supplies
- the overall 'state' of the working environment.

Contextual factors are mainly focused on the perceptions, beliefs, intentions and values of those involved and the meaning that they formulate and assign to the specific incident being analysed. These behaviour or motivational factors are not always observable or obvious. Examples that may be worth exploring include:

- what those involved believe to have actually happened at the time
- awareness of what they think is expected of them by the organisation, including meeting targets and following procedures
- awareness of specific work-based issues such as a tendency to disregard guidance because it was not generally trusted or was known to be out-of-date
- knowledge, or otherwise, of hazardous issues and other risks that are now only apparent to others.

Seek to Understand 'Local Rationality' – Why Decisions Made Sense

When looking back, it is essential to understand that ambulance clinicians and control staff make decisions with the goal of achieving success for patients and others. It needs to be recognised that this decision making (however 'strange' it seems to you and colleagues) made sense at the time to those involved. Their decisions or actions may have been based on incomplete or misleading information that was available, in addition to the overall frontline context and challenges that were experienced at that time. When reflecting on events retrospectively it is tempting to presume that all the information available now was available when the event occurred or was set in motion. Parking your hindsight bias at the door and exploring these decisions sensitively (and with learning in mind) with those involved, and others who have comparable work experiences, can be useful in better understanding these dynamic work situations and why things normally go right most of the time but sometimes go wrong.

Look 'Up and Out' Rather than 'Down and In'

Once different system factors and perspectives are identified, think about how these issues combined and interacted to contribute to both the immediate event and any similar past events that colleagues may recall – this provides a wider 'window on the system' (Vincent, 2004). Looking 'up and out' rather than 'down and in' focuses attention on broader system elements (Goode et al, 2018), including understanding how individual performances varied and were influenced by these factors, rather than simply focusing on individual behaviours which inevitably leads to a conclusion of 'human error' and all that this entails. Predictably, actions for improvement agreed in these circumstances may involve very limited and unsustainable solutions such as 'trying harder', 'more training' or incomplete learning such as 'better awareness', which may, albeit unintentionally, infer blame and appear punitive.

> **Box 10.1 – 'People Like Us'**
>
> An area of paramedic practice that may benefit from these principles of systems thinking is in relation to learning from complaints. The People Like Us report (2017) explored the nature of fitness to practise complaints made to the Health and Care Professions Council (HCPC) about paramedics, to consider why the number of complaints made in the paramedic profession were disproportionately higher in comparison to other HCPC healthcare professions.
>
> Several system elements such as public and societal expectations, the evolving nature of the profession, challenging practice and pressurised work environments were all highlighted as key influencing factors in the report. The review concluded that the perception that complaints to the regulator are only related to individual paramedics who are exceptions is not accurate for the majority of cases. Instead, most are 'people like us', where it was recognised that everyone – professionals, employers, professional bodies and regulators have a role to play in learning from complaints, rather than adopting a person-centred approach that focuses only on what the paramedic needs to learn.

Linear Thinking and Methods Limitations

Think carefully about the use of simple, linear 'cause and effect' methods to aid the analysis process where complex issues are concerned, as these are likely to have a limited and even misleading learning impact (Peerally et al, 2017). These approaches assume that things go wrong in the workplace because of a series of small '... events which interact sequentially with each other in a linear fashion and thus accidents are preventable by eliminating one of the causes in the linear sequence' (Health and

Chapter 10 – Learning from Events

Safety Professionals Alliance, 2012). For example, linear techniques such as Toyoda's 'Five Whys' (which appear to be in common usage in healthcare) involve a search for the 'root cause' of an event (Ohno, 1998). This may be suitable for identifying a production defect in a car manufacturing process, but potentially misguided in a highly complex and dynamically interacting system, such as in healthcare. Despite suggestions that these types of reviews should explore for 'root causes' (plural), they tend to focus on single system elements, rather than the multiple interactions between elements. Therefore, the relevance and application of these types of methods and the concept of 'root cause(s)' are now being questioned (Card, 2017; Peerally et al, 2017).

Learning from Events

Balancing Safety-I and Safety-II thinking

Traditionally, ambulance services have looked to what went wrong when trying to learn. In this type of Safety-I thinking (introduced in Chapter 1), safety is defined almost completely by *the absence of something*; the point where as few things as possible go wrong. This is achieved precisely by reduction – examining these 'wrong things' and repairing them. Safety-II aims to increase safety by maximising the number of events with a successful outcome. This means the unit of analysis goes beyond adverse events to studying how things happen under different conditions. This leads to an appreciation of system complexity that may improve incident investigation and quality improvement efforts, allowing development of more relevant prospective methods to improve safety (Hollnagel, 2014). A comparison of thinking between Safety-I and Safety-II is presented in Table 10.1.

Table 10.1 – Comparison of Safety-I and Safety-II thinking

Aspect	Safety-I	Safety-II
Definition of safety	Absence of adverse outcomes, absence of unacceptable levels of risk	Things going right, presence of resilience abilities
Safety management principle	Reactive following incidents, risk-based, control of risk through barriers	Proactive, continuously anticipating changes, achieving success through trade-offs and adaptation
Learning from experience	Learning from incidents and adverse outcomes, focus on root causes and contributory factors	Learning from everyday clinical work, focus on understanding work-as-done and trade-offs
Performance variability	Potentially harmful, constraining performance variability through standardisation and procedures	Inevitable and useful, source of success and failure

Source: Adapted from Hollnagel, 2014; Sujan, 2018

Although adverse events are not uncommon, it is still true that things usually go right for the vast majority of healthcare provided. Understanding why they usually go right may allow us to learn more, or different things about our complex systems. The Safety-II approach does not advocate that there is an abandonment of such Safety-I mechanisms for learning and promoting patient safety, but rather it emphasises how important it is to ensure that we apply systems thinking principles to the way that these are managed, maintained and further iterated and developed through co-production.

In Safety-II thinking, 'safety is defined as an ability – to make dynamic trade-offs and to adjust performance in order to meet changing demands and to deal with disturbances and surprises' (Sujan et al, 2017b). It may seem radical and even counterfactual but in practical terms care teams may 'improve their ability to learn from past experience by studying not only what goes wrong (i.e. incidents), but also by considering what goes right, i.e. by learning from everyday clinical work' (Sujan et al, 2017b). Identifying these types of situations and incorporating them into routine team-based meetings to enhance learning about care systems is one way of embedding Safety-II thinking. Another way is to ask, 'why do things normally go right?' before analysing why something went wrong.

Limitations of 'Never Event' Lists

There is growing interest in the 'never event' concept in international healthcare settings (de Wet et al, 2014; Department of Health, 2015), including ambulance organisations. These events refer to a subgroup of rare but serious patient safety incidents that are judged to be 'avoidable'. Lists of 'never events' have been formally included in adverse event review policies and processes (NHS Improvement, 2018). These cover a range of events, predominantly in hospital environments. Examples include wrong site surgery, retention of a foreign object after surgical procedure, incorrect medication administration, and undetected oesophageal intubation. Ambulance services are obviously aware of these lists, and understandably look to identify 'never events' that are specific to pre-hospital care. It can be difficult to agree an evidence-based list of pre-hospital 'never events', although we can find the term and some examples – such as unidentified accidental closure of an emergency call, hospital handover delay, ambulance wheel loss, and unrecognised misplaced endotracheal tube – in some UK ambulance service policies.

However, issues have been raised regarding the well-intentioned coupling of 'preventable harm' with zero tolerance 'never events', especially around the lack of evidence for such harm ever being totally preventable (Perrow, 1984; Zwetsloot et al, 2012; Waterson, 2017).

First, 'preventable' is logically derived from single case reviews, where decisions are made as to whether harm could have been prevented, i.e. the harm was not inevitable given patient acuity, medical knowledge and treatment available, and so on. However, at the statistical, patterned level, there is little or no evidence for such harm ever being preventable. Re-occurrence of most, if not all the types of harm is repeatedly observed (Attenello et al, 2015).

Chapter 10 – Learning from Events

Second, 'never event' is an emotive term about a narrower set of harm events, but it is important to stress that, while uncommon, they do occur with continuing regular frequency. This is demonstrated through reported data, such as the 435 incidents that were judged to have met the criteria of a 'never event' in NHS England between 1st of April 2019 and 29th of February 2020 (NHS Improvement, 2020).

The challenge for ambulance services is to consider whether the ideal of reducing preventable harm to 'never' is better for patient safety than, for example, the goal of managing risk materialising into harm to 'as low as reasonably practicable' (ALARP), which is well-established in other complex socio-technical systems and is demonstrably achievable (Sujan et al, 2017a). Alternative safety management strategies can be useful in understanding organisational risk related to the occurrence of such rare but serious events, for example: balancing Safety-I and Safety-II thinking and approaches (Hollnagel, 2014); the use of Safety Cases (The Health Foundation, 2012); barrier management principles and proactive methods such as Bowtie Analysis (McLeod and Bowie, 2018).

The 'never event' concept is well-intentioned but ultimately aspirational in a complex healthcare system. However, the way we think about patient safety is too important not to question assumptions and the potential implications of the various ways in which measured accountability might further its aims.

Implement Improvements to Enhance Care System Resilience

When first deciding whether changes for improvement are actually necessary as part of the event analysis, it may be wise to reflect on the following question: *What does normal care typically look like in this particular case?* If you find that an unprecedented event is extremely unlikely to re-occur in the same way, or that very minimal or no change is actually necessary, then 'be brave' and justify the need for no action based on the perceived (very low) risk of the event happening again, or having a similar impact if it does re-occur.

In terms of system improvement, it is likely that the care team will agree that multiple actions for improvement are necessary. However, it may not be feasible to consider and implement all of them; for instance, some recommendations may not fall within the remit or decision-making authority of the team. In this circumstance, identified improvement actions should be prioritised based on their perceived risk as a contributory factor to the future re-occurrence of the event, and what is feasible for the care team to implement taking into account available resources such as time, staffing and funding. In essence, care teams may have to perform 'trade-offs' (refer back to Chapter 4) between thoroughness and efficiency as part of their devised strategy to optimise improvement solutions and minimise the risk of event re-occurrence, or its consequences, if it does happen again.

Bear in mind that focusing on perceived easy 'fixes' – which rely on human behaviours such as recommending additional or refresher training for staff or issuing reminders to take specific actions at certain times – are likely to have limited impacts

> **Box 10.2 – Suggested Questions to Guide the Care Team when Considering Improvement Action**
>
> - Based on our analysis of what 'caused' the event, what should we do differently if and when a similar situation arises in the future?
> - Do we all agree that this is what we will do differently?
> - What can we do to ensure that we will remember this learning down the road?
> - If we are not the ones to implement this specific solution, how do we communicate this solution to the people who will be implementing it?
> - How sure are we that if a similar situation were to come up, we (or someone else) will respond appropriately?
>
> *Source:* Macrae (2014)

(Dekker, 2006). There is a greater chance for improvement to take hold if the full input and acceptance of all relevant staff has been obtained – for example, if a specific system of work is re-designed or a new technology is introduced. In other words, risk is more likely to be minimised when processes, systems and equipment are designed to accommodate the needs and capabilities of the people using them, rather than relying on people to change their behaviours to accommodate the system, as previously discussed in Chapter 5. The 'litmus test' in terms of improvement is always focused on whether the actions to be implemented will minimise the risk of event re-occurrence and its impacts. Questions to guide care teams when considering improvement actions are outlined in Box 10.2.

Summary

At its core, learning from events is based on sound educational principles and benefits significantly from a systems approach to more effectively reduce the risk of focusing on person-level issues, thereby enhancing insights, learning and potential design solutions. It is one key element among others in a 'learning organisation' that promotes an effective safety culture within care teams and organisations, and facilitates potential change for improvement. Importantly, the approach encourages a culture of honesty in the team as well as both individual and team-based reflection.

However, to make the process a much more meaningful experience, a deeper consideration of the emotional demands involved in highlighting an event (at the individual level) and the most professionally appropriate and effective way to analyse the event (at the team or organisational level) is required (Scott et al, 2009). Guiding the analysis using a basic HF/E framework can depersonalise the incident and focus attention on system-wide interacting contributory factors; that is, how the complexity of tasks, processes, technology and wider organisational issues can combine to increase the risk of things going wrong.

Chapter 10 – Learning from Events

A variation of team-based learning from events is established in other out-of-hospital care settings, such as in general medical practice, community pharmacy and primary care dentistry (Bowie et al, 2008). The challenge for ambulance service leaders and managers is how to translate such an approach to exploring and learning from safety incidents at the individual and team levels in the context of their settings. The reporting of safety-related incidents is potentially feasible for many given the right organisational and cultural conditions; however, deeper learning and meaningful action for improvement comes from the opportunity to reflect on such cases with peers in the spirit of learning, free from blame and potential punitive action. What needs to be done to enable this approach in ambulance services and paramedic practice?

References

Anderson, J.E., Kodate, N. (2015). Learning from patient safety incidents in incident review meetings: Organisational factors and indicators of analytic process effectiveness. *Safety Science*. 80: 105–114.

Attenello, F.J. et al. (2015). Incidence of 'never events' among weekend admissions versus weekday admissions to US hospitals: national analysis. *British Medical Journal*. 350:h1460.

Bowie, P. et al. (2005). A qualitative study of why general practitioners may participate in significant event analysis and educational peer review. *Quality & Safety in Health Care*. 14(3): 185–189.

Bowie, P., Pope, L., Lough, M. (2008). A review of the current evidence base for significant event analysis. *Journal of Evaluation in Clinical Practice*. 14(4): 520–536.

Braithwaite, J., Wears, R., Hollnagel, E. (2015). Resilient health care: turning patient safety on its head. *International Journal for Quality in Health Care*. 27: 418–420.

Card, A.J. (2017). The problem with five-whys. *BMJ Quality & Safety*. 26: 671–677.

Cook, R.I., Woods, D.D., Miller, C. (1998). A Tale of Two Stories: contrasting views of patient safety. Report from a workshop on assembling the scientific basis for progress on patient safety [online]. Available from: https://www.researchgate.net/publication/245102691_A_Tale_of_Two_Stories_Contrasting_Views_of_Patient_Safety

Dekker, S. (2006). *The Field Guide to Understanding Human Error*. Aldershot: Ashgate.

Dekker, S. (2013). *Second Victim: Error, Guilt, Trauma, and Resilience*. Boca Raton: CRC Press.

Department of Health (2015). *The Never Events Policy Framework: An update to the never events policy*. London: The Stationery Office.

de Wet, C. et al. (2014). Developing a preliminary 'never event' list for general practice using consensus-building methods. *British Journal of General Practice*. 64(620): 159–167.

Drupsteen, L., Groeneweg, J., Zwetsloot, G.I. (2013). Critical steps in learning from incidents: using learning potential in the process from reporting an incident to accident prevention. *International Journal of Occupational Safety and Ergonomics*. 19: 63–77.

Edmondson, A.C. et al. (2016). Understanding psychological safety in health care and education organizations: a comparative perspective. *Research in Human Development*. 13(1): 65–83.

Fisher, J.D. et al. (2015). Patient safety in ambulance services: a scoping review. *Health Services and Delivery Research*. 3(21).

Goode, N. et al. (2018). *Translating Systems Thinking into Practice: A guide to developing incident reporting systems*. Boca Raton: CRC Press.

Health and Safety Professionals Alliance (HaSPA) (2012). *The Core Body of Knowledge for Generalist OHS Professionals*. Tullamarine, VIC: Safety Institute of Australia.

References

Hollnagel, E. (2014). *Safety-I and Safety-II: the past and future of safety management*. Surrey: Ashgate.

Hollnagel, E., Wears, R.L., Braithwaite, J. (2015). From Safety-I to Safety-II: A White Paper. The Resilient Health Care Net: Published simultaneously by the University of Southern Denmark, University of Florida, USA, and Macquarie University, Australia. Available from: https://www.england.nhs.uk/signuptosafety/wp-content/uploads/sites/16/2015/10/safety-1-safety-2-whte-papr.pdf

Hulme, A. et al. (2019). What do applications of systems thinking accident analysis methods tell us about accident causation? A systematic review of applications between 1990 and 2018. *Safety Science*. 117: 164–183.

Macrae, C. (2014). *Close Calls: Managing Risk and Resilience in Airline Flight Safety*. London: Palgrave.

Macrae, C. (2016). The problem with incident reporting. *BMJ Quality & Safety*. 25: 71–75.

McKay, J. et al. (2009). A review of significant events analysed in general medical practice: implications for the quality and safety of patient care. *BMC Family Practice*. 10: 61.

McLeod, R.W., Bowie, P. (2018). Bowtie Analysis as a prospective risk assessment technique in primary healthcare. *Policy and Practice in Health and Safety*. 16(2): 177–193.

McNab, D. et al. (2016). Understanding and responding when things go wrong: key principles for primary care educators. *Education for Primary Care*. 27: 258–266.

NHS Improvement (2018). Never Events list 2018 [online]. Available from: https://improvement.nhs.uk/documents/2266/Never_Events_list_2018_FINAL_v5.pdf

NHS Improvement (2020). Provisional publication of Never Events reported as occurring between 1 April 2019 and 29 February 2020 [online]. Available from: https://improvement.nhs.uk/documents/6584/Provisional_publication_-_NE_1_April_2019_-_29_February_2020.pdf

Ohno, T. (1998). *Toyota Production System: Beyond Large-Scale Production*. Portland: Productivity Press.

Ozeke, O. et al. (2019). Second victims in health care: current perspectives. *Advances in Medical Education and Practice*. 10: 593–603.

Peerally, M.F. et al. (2017). The problem with root cause analysis. *BMJ Quality & Safety*. 26: 417–422.

Perrow, C. (1984). *Normal Accidents*. New Jersey: Princeton University Press.

Pringle, M. et al. (1995). Significant event auditing: a study of the feasibility and potential of case-based auditing in primary medical care. *Occasional Paper Series (Royal College of General Practitioners)*. March (70): 1–21.

Rasmussen, J. (1997). Risk management in a dynamic society: a modelling problem. *Safety Science*. 27(2–3): 183–213.

Rasmussen, J., Svedung, I. (2000). Proactive Risk Management in a Dynamic Society. Statens räddningsverk (Swedish Rescue Services Agency), Sweden.

Scott, S.D. et al. (2009). The natural history of recovery for the healthcare provider 'second victim' after adverse patient events. *Quality & Safety in Health Care*. 18(5): 325–330.

Shojania, K. (2008). The frustrating case of incident reporting systems. *Quality & Safety in Health Care*. 17(6): 400–403.

Shorrock, S. (2017). Planes, Trains and Envelopes. Trent Simulation & Clinical Skills Centre [online]. Available from: https://www.youtube.com/watch?v=bQPCQqHkiVc

Sujan, M. (2018). A Safety-II perspective on organisational learning in healthcare organisations. *International Journal of Health Policy Management*. 7(7): 662–666.

Chapter 10 – Learning from Events

Sujan, M.A. et al. (2017a). How can health care organisations make and justify decisions about risk reduction? Lessons from a cross-industry review and a health care stakeholder consensus development process. *Reliability Engineering and System Safety*. 161: 1–11.

Sujan, M.A., Huang, H., Braithwaite, J. (2017b). Learning from incidents in health care: critique from a Safety-II perspective. *Safety Science*. 99: 115–121.

The Health Foundation (2012). Evidence: Using safety cases in industries and healthcare [online]. Available from: https://www.health.org.uk/sites/default/files/UsingSafetyCasesInIndustryAndHealthcare.pdf

Vincent, C. (2004). Analysis of clinical incidents: a window on the system not a search for root causes. *Quality & Safety in Health Care*. 13(4):242–243.

Waterson, P. (2017). That strange number 'zero'. *Policy and Practice in Health and Safety*. 15(2): 85–87.

Wu, A.W., Steckelberg, R.C. (2012). Medical error, incident investigation and the second victim: Doing better but feeling worse? *BMJ Quality & Safety*. 21(4): 267–270.

Zwetsloot, G.I.J.M. et al. (2013). The case for research into the zero accident vision. *Safety Science*. 58: 41–48.

Chapter 11
Safety Culture: Theory and Practice

Steven Shorrock and Paul Bowie

In this chapter:
- Theoretical concepts, definitions and differences of safety culture and safety climate
- Importance of exploring safety culture in ambulance services
- Barriers to reliably 'measuring' workforce perceptions of safety culture
- Introduction to discussion cards as a practical and meaningful approach to understanding aspects of safety culture

Introduction

To improve system performance and staff well-being, there needs to be a focus on the cultural context of work (Reason, 1998). The 'safety culture' within a healthcare team and organisation is an important public health concern internationally, including in pre-hospital care (Francis, 2013; Curran et al, 2018; Sørskår et al, 2019). While there is limited research and practice on safety culture in ambulance services, much can be learned from other high-risk industries and healthcare sectors on how safety is valued and prioritised by both frontline staff groups, managers and leaders (Marshall et al, 2003; WHO, 2009).

What is Meant by 'Safety Culture'?

Defining a concept such as safety culture is a subject of much debate (Hopkins, 2006). This is summed up in two humorous quotations from academic experts in the field. For James Reason, safety culture '… has all the definitional precision of a cloud' (Reason, 1997), while for Ken Catchpole, '… the idea of "culture" is perhaps similar to that of "intelligence" – everyone thinks they know what it is, but conceptual clarity is more elusive' (Catchpole, 2014).

Chapter 11 – Safety Culture: Theory and Practice

While there are many definitions of safety culture, most emphasise shared assumptions, values, beliefs and patterns of behaviour concerning safety. These tend to change very slowly and are likely to differ between work groups. But there is often confusion over the difference between the terms 'safety culture' and 'safety climate'. Although both terms are inextricably linked and often used interchangeably, they are different theoretical concepts (Cooper, 2000; Reason, 2008). Safety culture as a term was reportedly first coined in the investigation report into the Chernobyl nuclear accident, which suggested that organisations can reduce safety incidents and accidents if they build a 'positive safety culture' (The Health Foundation, 2011). A pragmatic view suggests that safety culture can be 'viewed as an enduring characteristic of an organisation' whereas safety climate can be thought of as a 'temporary state of an organisation that is subject to change' (Meyer and Reniers, 2016). Guldenmund (2014) agreed that 'safety climate is considered to be a transient psychological variable, much less stable than safety culture'. Climate might be said to be more akin to the mood of a group or organisation, while culture is more akin to its personality.

Importance of Safety Culture

There is wide agreement that safety culture is an important concept (Reason, 1998; Francis, 2013), as organisations with a positive safety culture are thought to be more likely to learn openly and effectively from failure and adapt their working practices appropriately (Cooper, 2000; Guldenmund, 2007). The converse is true for a weak safety culture, which has been implicated as a significant contributory factor in many catastrophic organisational incidents – for example, the Piper Alpha oil platform explosion, the Space Shuttle Challenger disaster and the Zeebrugge ferry incident (Reason, 2008). Comparable incidents in UK healthcare, where a poorly developed safety culture was cited as a contributory factor, would include the failings highlighted in Stafford Hospital (high mortality rates from emergency admissions; BBC, 2012; Francis, 2013) and Bristol Royal Infirmary (high infant surgical mortality rates; BBC, 2000) in England, and the Vale of Leven Hospital (deaths associated with *Clostridium difficile*; BBC, 2014) in Scotland. Most modern healthcare systems have therefore embraced the notion of building a positive safety culture, which has been reinforced in safety policies and as part of national improvement programmes. The challenge lies in how this can be achieved in everyday care work.

What the aforementioned major incidents have shown us is the influence of high-level organisational factors and design issues on safety performance and related failures, rather than much of the previous (simplistic) focus, especially in the media, on improving only local processes or eradicating frontline 'human error' issues (Wagenaar et al, 1990). It is only in more recent years that we have begun to look seriously at how we can understand safety culture in healthcare settings to identify related issues and consider their implications in relation to safer care.

In reviews of safety culture research (Cooper, 2000; Gadd and Collins, 2002), a number of organisational systems, behaviours and psychological attributes were identified that distinguished organisations with low accident or incident rates from

Importance of Safety Culture

those with higher rates. Examples with direct relevance to ambulance services include:

- strong senior management and leadership commitment and involvement in safety
- a mature, stable workforce
- good personnel selection and retention, job placement and promotion procedures
- good induction and follow-up safety training
- ongoing safety schemes reinforcing the importance of safety, including near-miss reporting
- accepting that promotion of a safety culture is a long-term strategy that requires sustained effort and interest
- thoroughly investigating all safety incidents and near misses
- regular auditing of safety systems to provide feedback on performance and ideas for improvement
- capturing attitudes towards incident reporting and analysis, job-induced stress and poor working conditions
- regularly assessing safety culture and improving safety behaviours.

Acting, where appropriate, on regular information from these activities combined with knowledge of what can go wrong can lead to the creation of an 'informed' safety culture. This is also the 'best way to stay cautious' about safety performance while taking 'a systematic approach to potentially predicting and preventing incidents' (Reason, 1998).

By exploring issues within groups such as paramedics and other ambulance service staff, we can begin to understand the contexts and situations in which undesirable (and desirable) safety-related issues can materialise (Cooper, 2000). Naturally, staff have both shared and different assumptions, attitudes and perspectives about work and safety. Problems tend to arise when assumptions remain below the surface, and when problematic consensus or conflict is not understood. Examples include assumptions and beliefs about how systems work, who performs which tasks, the complexity of those tasks, system safety and reliability, and about resourcing (Guldenmund, 2000). Additionally, different team members will be aware of recent incidents or existing system problems, risks and hazards, and daily work hassles that others do not know about. The related interactions between people and other elements of the system will also contribute to frustration, anxiety, stress and irritation in the workplace, which will impact human performance, and ultimately patient safety (Cooper, 2001; Flin et al, 2006). The evaluation of care team perceptions of the prevailing safety culture can shine a light on these types of issues by providing all staff with the opportunity to begin to explore how things *really* work in healthcare, including ambulance and paramedic services.

Chapter 11 – Safety Culture: Theory and Practice

Understanding Safety Culture

The perceived importance of safety culture in improving patient safety and its potential impact on other emergent system outcomes (such as staff well-being or patient experience) has led to a growing interest in attempting to understand the prevailing safety culture in organisations across most healthcare sectors worldwide (Waterson, 2014).

Guldenmund (2014) outlines three major approaches to understanding safety culture. The three approaches not only use different methods, but have different assumptions about the nature of culture, and therefore safety culture:

- The first is the *academic or anthropological approach*. This approach focuses on describing rather than evaluating, and is qualitative in nature, which may involve ethnography or case study, for example. Methods tend to involve interviews, observation and reviews of documents and other artefacts. Accordingly, the results are not 'measured' or 'quantified'.

- The second approach is the *analytical or psychological approach*. This approach focuses on measuring and evaluating. This typically involves the use of survey questionnaires that include concepts and factors thought – from prior research – to be pertinent to safety culture; what Guldenmund describes as a 'web of concepts'. Different organisations, or groups within organisations, are scored on these different culture concepts or factors (for example, perceptions of leadership or team working).

- The third approach is the *pragmatic or experience-based approach*. This approach is normative – what an organisation should do. The approach may involve descriptions of how a mature status may be obtained, for instance, via a 'ladder' approach with descriptive terms attached to each rung of the ladder (for example, pathological, bureaucratic and generative; Westrum, 2004). These descriptions and ratings of cultural maturity are normally done in groups.

Translating Safety Culture for Ambulance Services

In viewing safety culture within the context of pre-hospital settings, the underlying assumption is that it strongly influences clinicians and staff to choose behaviours that enhance – rather than compromise – prevailing safety practices and thinking. This poses an important question: can a healthcare organisation develop a safety culture that encourages this, and is capable of improving specific patient safety outcomes? Research suggests this is difficult and problematic, but this need not prevent organisations from taking on the challenge.

The first step involves a very basic requirement to actually explore and discuss the concept of a 'safety culture'. This implies that something as intangible, perhaps ethereal, can be adequately defined, understood, acted upon and improved by healthcare leaders, clinicians, managers and staff in the way that policymakers assume.

Translating Safety Culture for Ambulance Services

For pre-hospital care settings, therefore, the big challenge is to think more critically about how organisations perceive and approach issues of patient safety and improvement, and perhaps draw some inspiration from the principles, ideas and multiple methods outlined in this book. It is important to recognise that the leadership commitment to patient safety within a service organisation is strongly linked to the maturity level of the prevailing safety culture. The organisational leadership strongly influences the necessary workplace culture to ensure that patient safety and care improvement are valued as 'everybody's business' (Apekey et al, 2011).

Establishing a 'just culture' that enables the whole team to support and advance patient safety is, therefore, only possible with strong leadership support and action (Table 11.1). It is for the organisation to facilitate and build a culture of trust that encourages, for example, effective team working, collective learning from safety incidents and strong communication across and beyond the organisation. They have both the responsibility and the authority to ensure that there is a continued focus on

Table 11.1 – Leadership influence on types of safety culture

Element of Safety Culture	Characteristics
Open culture	Staff feel comfortable discussing patient safety incidents and raising safety issues with both colleagues and senior staff
Just culture	Staff, patients and carers are treated fairly, with empathy and consideration when they have been involved in a patient safety incident or have raised a safety issue
Reporting culture	Staff have confidence in the local incident reporting system and use it to notify healthcare managers of incidents that are occurring, including near misses. Barriers to incident reporting have been identified and removed: • staff are not blamed and punished when they report incidents • they receive constructive feedback after submitting an incident report • the reporting process itself is easy
Learning culture	The organisation: • is committed to learning safety lessons • communicates them to colleagues • remembers them over time
Informed culture	The organisation has learned from past experience and has the ability to identify and mitigate future incidents, because it learns from events that have already happened (e.g. incident reports, investigations and why things generally go well)

Source: Patient Safety First (2009)

Chapter 11 – Safety Culture: Theory and Practice

improving the safety of patient care – in essence, establishing safety as a cultural 'value' as well as a service 'priority', and creating the conditions for related learning and action for improvement.

The Problem with 'Measuring' Safety Culture

The bulk of safety culture research and practice is driven by measurement methods such as survey questionnaires associated with analytical approaches. This has a number of problems. For instance, from an anthropological perspective, culture cannot be analysed into constituent concepts or factors, and cannot be quantified. Even if these analytical assumptions were valid, the average of scores does not necessarily quantify a culture, and any data are ordinal, meaning that different scores for different groups (or over time) may indicate no more than 'greater than' or 'less than'; it cannot be assumed that there are equal intervals between values on a scale (for example, 1 to 5). Questionnaires are also thought to access the more superficial aspects of values, attitudes and beliefs, which accords more with 'safety climate'. However, as previously mentioned, the terms 'safety culture' and 'safety climate' are commonly used interchangeably in the literature (Mearns and Flin, 1996).

There are currently hundreds of different questionnaires that have been specially adapted, developed and tested for healthcare, including a small number specifically for pre-hospital care. However, the rigour with which such safety climate tools are psychometrically designed and tested was shown to be highly variable in an early study published by Flin and colleagues (Flin et al, 2006), and is still the same over a decade on (Al Salem et al, 2019). This recent systematic review of questionnaire studies of safety climate in acute hospital settings by Al Salem and colleagues included only five such questionnaire tools, demonstrating very limited progress. Detailed inspection of each study revealed ambiguity around concepts of safety culture and climate, safety climate dimensions, and problems with the design of these measures. The review concluded that evidence of the adequacy of the psychometric development of safety climate questionnaire tools is still very limited. It recommended research to resolve the controversies in the definitions and dimensions of safety culture and climate in healthcare, and in the validation of safety climate questionnaires.

Let's take a real example in another care setting to illustrate this problematic measurement issue. Figure 11.1 depicts a high-level summary of national data from surveys of safety climate perceptions among the Scottish general medical practice workforce in 2014 and 2015 (MacWalter et al, 2019). The survey used a questionnaire tool co-designed and validated with users (de Wet et al, 2010), and with 'gold standard' psychometric properties as reported in a recent systematic review (Curran et al, 2018). Excellent response rates of greater than 90% were achieved in each year, possibly as a result of participation being financially incentivised as part of service contract obligations.

While the results of the survey indicate trend-type information overall, it could be argued to be of limited value, as are the findings reported for each of the domains.

The Problem with 'Measuring' Safety Culture

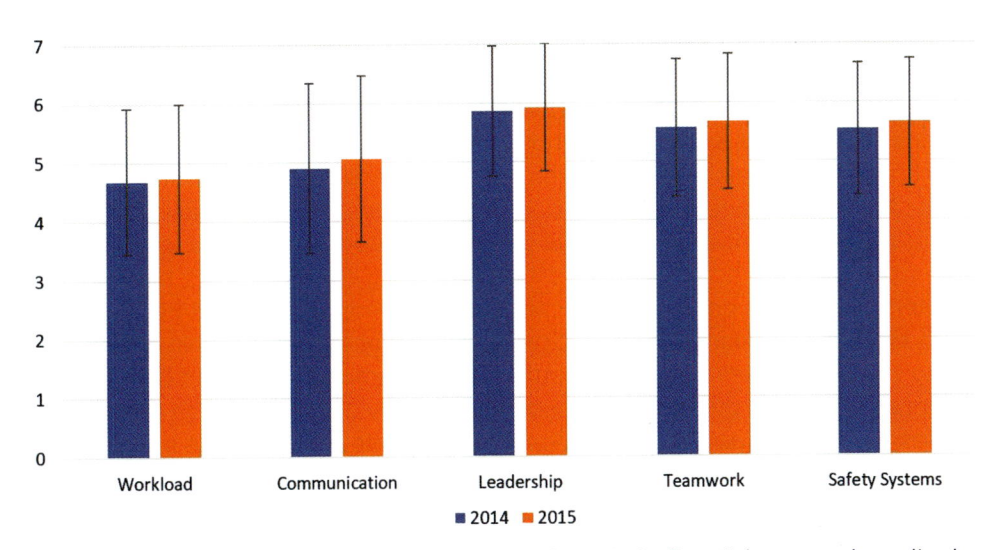

Figure 11.1 – Survey scores by safety climate domain in Scottish general medical practice
Note: 7-point Likert scale – a higher score indicates a more positive climate domain perception
Source: Adapted from MacWalter et al (2019)

Yes, we can see that workload and communication issues score noticeably lower than the other domains across both survey periods and that this might be of general interest to national policy makers, politicians and executive leaders, for example. But how does this translate into something that is practically meaningful for healthcare organisations and teams in a way that drives learning and improvements in system performance? The development, implementation and evaluation of these types of surveys take up significant resources, energy and time. The question is, is it really contributing to organisational learning and improvement as much as anticipated, or in the way that is desired? This is particularly pertinent because we cannot reliably associate (or correlate) the results with clinical or organisational outcomes – the 'holy grail' of safety culture measurement (Al Salem et al, 2019), at least in general practice. Given the limitations of the evidence base it is difficult to agree on the benefits of 'survey measurement' in terms of organisational learning.

Another problem with safety culture measurement is that it is essentially a top-down activity. From experience, the results can tend to be reduced to quantitative scores, which become of particular interest to managers, who naturally wish to see the scores improve. This sometimes involves attaching performance targets or incentives to the scores, and this may lead to unintended consequences, such as direct focus on the scores and resultant short-term actions to influence them, rather than understanding and tackling the wider issues. Furthermore, the attempts at measurement and intervention are usually controlled and conducted far away from the frontline staff groups, by researchers or consultants, for instance, with the results delivered to management. This has been described as 'done to' and 'done for' instead of 'done with' and 'done by' (Russell, 2019).

Chapter 11 – Safety Culture: Theory and Practice

Translating Theory into Practice

Now that we have examined the limitations of safety climate survey tools, how can we meaningfully reflect on the concept of safety culture and what can be done in practice? Translating safety culture theory into a practical educational intervention that has utility for frontline care teams and organisations (beyond feedback from related ad hoc questionnaire surveys) is clearly a challenge. However, a format used in other work and healthcare settings is that of 'playing cards'. This has been used in the context of drug use and harm reduction (London Drug and Alcohol Policy Forum, 2020) and design ('Design with Intent Cards', Lockton et al, 2010). Within the area of safety culture, The Keil Centre (a Scottish-based Human Factors and Ergonomics consultancy) also uses a card-sorting approach to provide an indication of an organisation's maturity, with each element of safety culture having five maturity levels.

Taking inspiration from such approaches, EUROCONTROL (an intergovernmental organisation for air traffic management across Europe) designed Safety Culture Discussion Cards to provide a practical resource for teams to use themselves, without the need for external support. The approach grew from the EUROCONTROL Safety Culture programme, which involves questionnaires, focus groups and interviews, spanning over 30 countries (see Shorrock et al 2011; Kirwan and Shorrock, 2014). The aim of the cards was to provide a resource to aid discussion about safety culture by any person or team, including staff and managers in air traffic operations, maintenance, specialist and support staff (such as safety, quality, projects, human resources, legal) (Shorrock, 2012). To address this aim, several requirements were specified to ensure the discussion cards were useful:

- First, the cards should be **engaging**. The cards are not a tool for 'experts' and should not be perceived as such (though they may be used by safety and human factors specialists). Rather, they are a tool for any individual or group who wishes to use them. They should therefore promote ownership and provoke discussion.

- Second, the cards should be **educational**. The potential audience will know little about the theory of safety culture and have only a lay understanding of the possible issues. Frontline professionals (such as air traffic controllers or maintenance technicians in the EUROCONTROL context) often have a sharper understanding of some aspects of safety culture from their operational experience, so the cards need also to build on this.

- Third, the cards should be **flexible**. Inherent in the concept of a regular pack of cards is that there are several possible 'games' or uses. Similarly, no particular 'method' is prescribed for the Safety Culture Discussion Cards. Rather, several options are described as possible uses, but participants may use the cards however they wish. To enhance flexibility, the cards should be a physical product, but may also be used digitally, for instance, on smartphones.

- Fourth, the content, especially the headlines and pictures, should be **memorable**. If users can recognise or even recall aspects of the cards when they are not using them, this will aid the educational value and usefulness. This requires that the cards are distinctive and attractive.

- Fifth, the cards should have an acceptable degree of **validity** – both theoretical and practical. While the cards are a heuristic tool rather than a method for measurement, they should be based on a theoretical model of safety culture and represent a comprehensive range of issues.

- Finally, and most importantly, the cards should be **useful**. They should ultimately help the users to think of ways to improve safety culture – and inspire them to take action based on the results. Many of these requirements involve bridging the gap between research and practice (Chung and Shorrock, 2011), translating research-based concepts and putting them into the hands of paramedics and ambulance staff.

Development of Health and Social Care Safety Culture Discussion Cards

In 2018, the safety, skills and improvement research team at NHS Education for Scotland (the main education and training body for the healthcare workforce) worked on a participatory design basis with a range of clinicians and managers to adapt the EUROCONTROL Safety Culture Discussion Cards for generic use by any health and social care team. This largely involved making minor changes in terminology to make the language used in the cards more relevant and accessible to health and social care teams and work contexts. Since the cards are intended for use by potentially anybody within these settings, the design elements had to strike a balance on several levels, for instance, guiding without being patronising, challenging without being confrontational. The cards are now used by many different care teams across the UK as well as in Canada and New Zealand.

The pack of discussion cards (Figure 11.2) comprises the following:

- **Front card** – the first card is analogous to a book cover for the set of cards.
- **What is safety culture?** – a single card is used to provide a simple definition of safety culture and its importance for safety.
- **Organisation of the cards** – the EUROCONTROL safety culture elements provide the structure for the cards.
- **How to use these cards** – several cards are used to provide ideas for how the cards might be used. The options described include the following:
    - Comparing views: Different members of a team or different teams sort the cards into two piles: 'What we do well' and 'What we need to improve', then compare and discuss the piles.
    - Safety moments: In a small group, the users take just one card and discuss the card for 10–15 minutes, taking brief notes of any actions arising from the discussion.

Chapter 11 – Safety Culture: Theory and Practice

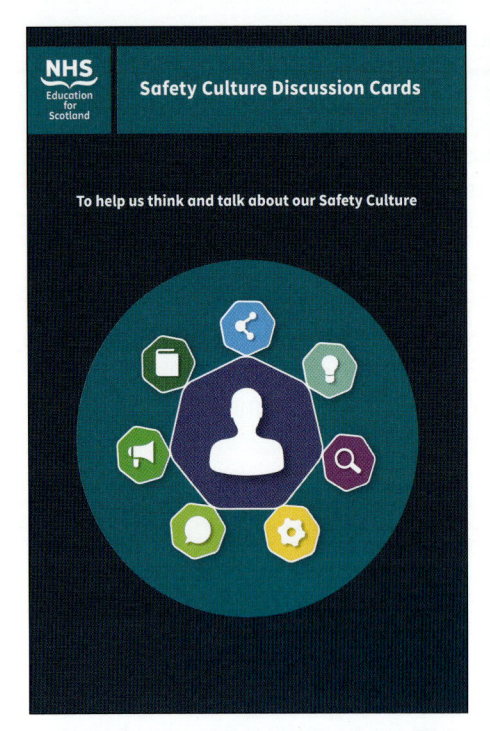

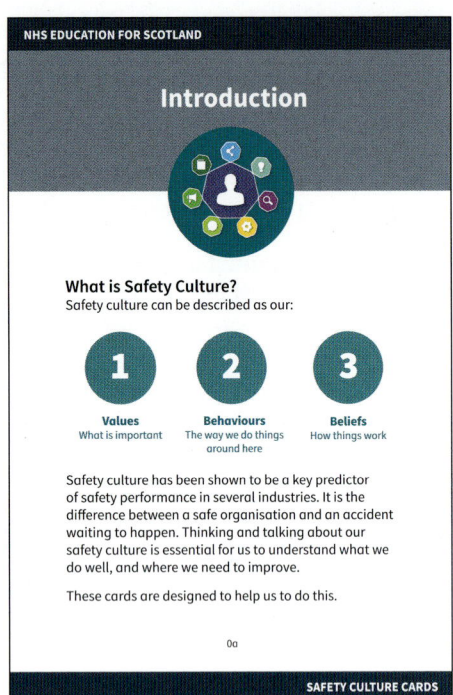

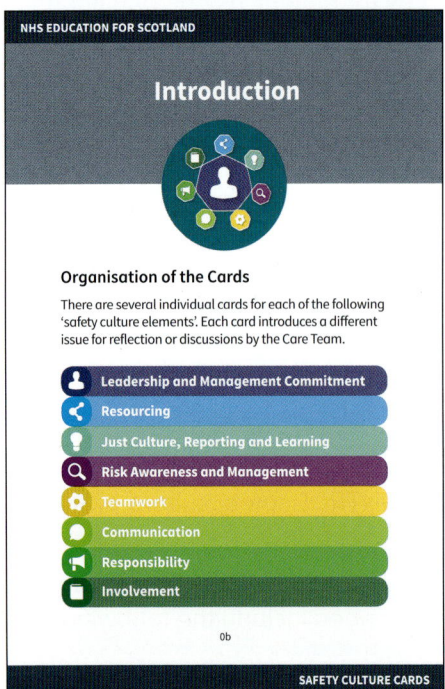

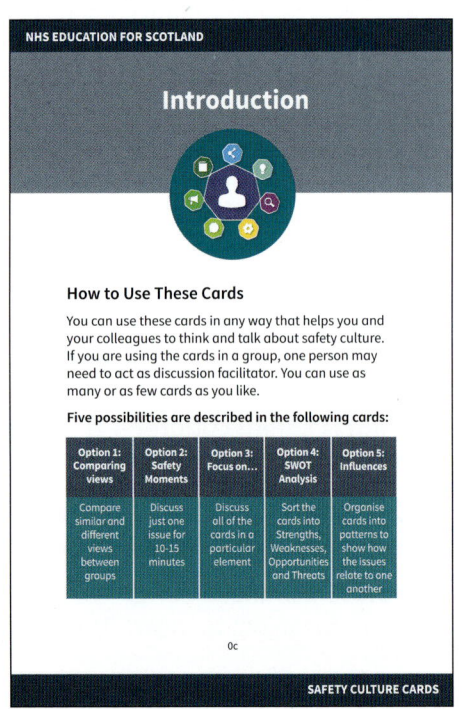

Figure 11.2 – Examples of the NHS Education for Scotland Safety Culture Discussion Cards for Health and Social Care Teams

Source: NHS Education for Scotland (2018). Reproduced with permission

Development of Health and Social Care Safety Culture Discussion Cards

NHS EDUCATION FOR SCOTLAND

Introduction

Option 1: Comparing Views

Different members of your team can sort cards into 2 piles: what we do well and what we need to improve (your 'team' may be your organisation unit, professional group, etc):

What we do well & what we need to improve

Then compare the piles and discuss:
- Where do we agree?
- Where do we disagree?
- What are the priority issues to address?
- What might happen if they are not addressed?
- How can this be done?
- Who needs to be involved (responsible, consulted, informed)?
- When does it need to be done?

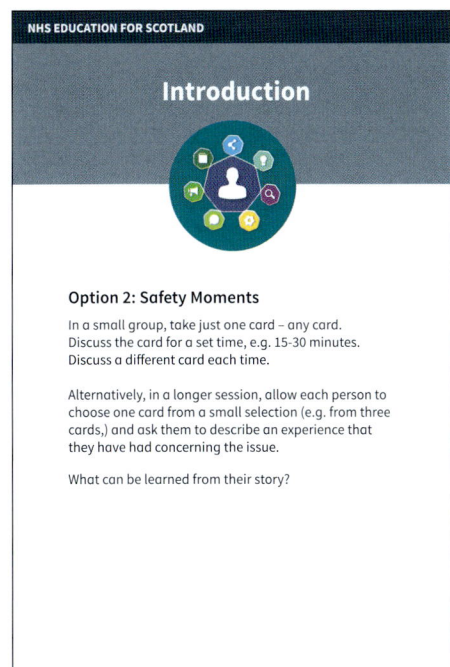

NHS EDUCATION FOR SCOTLAND

Introduction

Option 2: Safety Moments

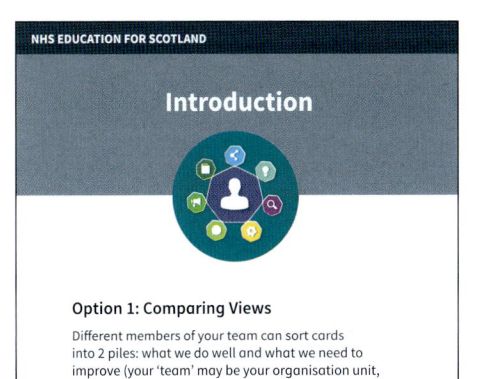

In a small group, take just one card – any card. Discuss the card for a set time, e.g. 15-30 minutes. Discuss a different card each time.

Alternatively, in a longer session, allow each person to choose one card from a small selection (e.g. from three cards,) and ask them to describe an experience that they have had concerning the issue.

What can be learned from their story?

NHS EDUCATION FOR SCOTLAND

Introduction

Option 3: Focus on…

Choose a specific element, such as 'Resourcing', and discuss each card in depth with your colleagues.

You may sort the cards or consider questions such as:
- What do we do well?
- What and where is our 'best practice' on this issue?
- Where have we improved?
- Where do we need to improve?
- What are we avoiding… where are our 'blindspots'?
- What is stopping us from improving?
- How can we improve the situation?

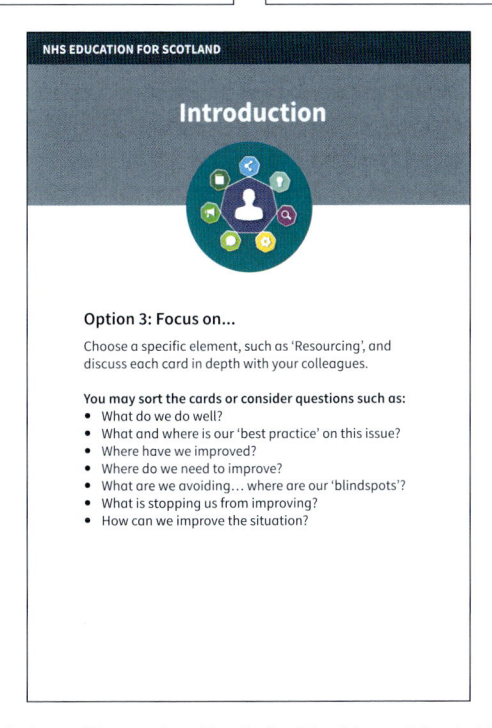

A PDF copy of the Safety Culture Discussion Cards for Health and Social Care Teams can be freely downloaded here: https://learn.nes.nhs.scot/6036/patient-safety-zone/primary-care-patient-safety-resources/safety-culture-discussion-cards.

Chapter 11 – Safety Culture: Theory and Practice

- ■ Focus on...: The users choose a specific element, such as 'Resourcing', and discuss each card in depth with their colleagues. Users may sort the cards or consider questions such as: What do we do well? What and where is our 'best practice' on this issue? Where do we need to improve?
- ■ SWOT analysis: The users sort the cards into strengths, weaknesses, opportunities and threats, and discuss the results.
- **Discussion cards** – the discussion cards are sorted into eight elements of relevance to safety culture: Leadership and management commitment; Resourcing; Just culture, reporting and learning; Risk awareness and management; Teamwork; Communication; Responsibility; and Involvement. There are several cards in each element.

Each discussion card shares a common formula in terms of design elements:

- **Headline** – each card has one or a few words to characterise the issue. Some of these are phrased directly as 'good practice' (for example, 'Avoid the blame game'; 'Challenge risk'; 'Speak up'). Others are phrased more indirectly where such a direct phrasing could be considered patronising or affected. Concrete examples include 'Teamwork on the front line' and 'Managing risk', while more abstract examples include 'Blind spots' (concerning risk awareness) and 'Going up, going down' (concerning vertical communication).
- **Question** – following the headline, a probing question is asked (a mix of open and closed questions) concerning the current situation.
- **Rationale** – following each statement is one or two sentences providing context or explanation for the question and headline. For the 'Blind spots' example, the rationale is 'Sometimes problems seem so long-standing or difficult to resolve that they are ignored and become a 'blind spot'.'
- **Follow-up question** – finally, a second question is asked, either probing the issue further, or asking how the situation could be improved, by the individual, the team or organisation. For the 'Blind spots' card, this is 'How can you help to make sure that safety problems are resolved rather than ignored?'

Summary

Defining and understanding 'safety culture', and influencing it is a big challenge for ambulance services. However, the theoretical concept of safety culture and the practical use of discussion cards provide a means for paramedics, control centre staff, support staff, managers and leaders at all levels of ambulance services to discuss related concepts based on an established model and set of items. The real value of this approach is in encouraging ownership of concepts and cards, removing the perceived mystique and fuzziness of 'safety culture' and putting it back into the hands of those who are part of the culture.

The act of reflecting upon and discussing safety culture is relatively new to healthcare teams and more research, development and evaluation work are required to provide a better understanding of what a positive safety culture entails and how this can be further validated, particularly in pre-hospital care settings.

If the mismatch between healthcare policy rhetoric (work-as-imagined) and sharp-end reality (work-as-done) is to be reduced, and if patient safety is to be improved, then pre-hospital organisations should focus on providing protected time for paramedics, ambulance control centre staff and other care team members to better understand safety in the context of everyday safety work.

References

Al Salem, G., Bowie, P., Morrison, J. (2019). Hospital survey on patient safety culture: psychometric evaluation in Kuwaiti public healthcare settings. *BMJ Open*. 9(5): e028666.

Apekey, T.A. et al. (2011). Room for improvement? Leadership, innovation culture and uptake of quality improvement methods in general practice. *Journal of Evaluation in Clinical Practice*. 17(2): 311–318.

BBC (2000). Bristol 'had double normal death rates'. 29th September 2000 [online]. http://news.bbc.co.uk/1/hi/health/947204.stm.

BBC (2012). Stafford Hospital reports serious patient safety breaches. 26th January 2012 [online]. https://www.bbc.co.uk/news/uk-england-stoke-staffordshire-16736694.

BBC (2014). Vale of Leven C. diff inquiry criticises health board. 24th November 2014 [online]. https://www.bbc.co.uk/news/uk-scotland-glasgow-west-30150343.

Catchpole, K. (2014). Foreword. In: Waterson, P. (ed.). *Patient Safety Culture: Theory, methods and application*. Farnham: Ashgate. pp. xxiii–xxvi.

Chung, A.Z.Q., Shorrock, S.T. (2011). The research–practice relationship in ergonomics and human factors – surveying and bridging the gap. *Ergonomics*. 54(5): 413–429.

Cooper, M.D. (2000). Towards a model of safety culture. *Safety Science*. 36(2): 111–136.

Cooper, M.D. (2001). Treating safety as a value. *Professional Safety*. 46(2): 17–21.

Curran, C. et al. (2018). A systematic review of primary care safety climate survey instruments: Their origins, psychometric properties, quality and usage. *Journal of Patient Safety*. 14(2): e9–e18.

Department of Health (2001). Doing Less Harm: Improving the safety and quality of care through reporting, analysing and learning from adverse incidents involving NHS patients – key requirements for healthcare providers. London: HMSO.

de Wet, C. et al. (2010). The development and psychometric evaluation of a safety climate measure for primary care. *Quality & Safety in Health Care*. 19(6): 578–584.

Flin, R. et al. (2006). Measuring safety climate in health care. *Quality & Safety in Health Care*. 15(2): 109–115.

Francis, R. (2013). *Report of the Mid Staffordshire NHS Foundation Trust Public Inquiry*. London: The Stationery Office.

Gadd, S., Collins, A.M. (2002). *Safety Culture: A review of the literature*. Report No. HSL/2002/25. Sheffield, UK: Health & Safety Laboratory.

Guldenmund, F.W. (2000). The nature of safety culture: a review of theory and research. *Safety Science*. 34: 215–257.

Guldenmund, F.W. (2007). The use of questionnaires in safety culture research and evaluation. *Safety Science*. 45: 723–743.

Guldenmund, F. (2014). Organisational safety culture principles. In: Waterson, P. (ed.). *Patient Safety Culture: Theory, methods and application*. Farnham: Ashgate, pp. 349–370.

Chapter 11 – Safety Culture: Theory and Practice

Hopkins, A. (2006). Studying organisational cultures and their effects on safety. *Safety Science*. 44: 875–889.

Kirwan, B., Shorrock, S. (2014). A view from elsewhere: safety culture in European air traffic management. In: Waterson, P. (ed.) *Patient Safety Culture: Theory, methods and application*. Farnham: Ashgate, pp. 349–370.

Lockton, D., Harrison, D., Stanton, N.A. (2010). *Design with Intent: 101 Patterns for Influencing Behaviour Through Design*.

London Drug and Alcohol Policy Forum (2020). Playing cards [online]. Available from: https://stage.cityoflondon.gov.uk/services/health-and-wellbeing/drugs-and-alcohol/london-drug-and-alcohol-policy-forum/Pages/playing-cards.aspx

MacWalter, G. et al. (2019). Measuring Safety Climate in Scottish General Practices. SKIRC Technical Report. Edinburgh [online]. Available from: https://www.researchgate.net/publication/332781842_Measuring_Safety_Climate_in_Scottish_General_Medical_Practices

Marshall, M. et al. (2003). Culture of safety. *Quality & Safety in Health Care*. 12(4): 318.

Mearns, K., Flin, R. (1996). Assessing the state of organizational safety – culture or climate? *Current Psychology*. 18(1): 5–17.

Meyer, T., Reniers, G. (2016). *Engineering Risk Management*. 2nd Ed. Berlin: De Gruyter.

NHS Education for Scotland (2018). Safety culture discussion cards. Available from: A PDF copy of the Safety Culture Discussion Cards for Health and Social Care Teams can be freely downloaded here: https://learn.nes.nhs.scot/6036/patient-safety-zone/primary-care-patient-safety-resources/safety-culture-discussion-cards.

Patient Safety First. (2009) The 'how to guide' for implementing human factors in healthcare [online]. Available from: https://chfg.org/how-to-guide-to-human-factors-volume-1/

Reason, J. (1997). *Managing the Risks of Organizational Accidents*. Aldershot: Ashgate.

Reason, J. (1998). Achieving a safe culture: theory and practice. *Work Stress*. 12(3): 293–306.

Reason, J. (2008). *The Human Contribution: Unsafe acts, accidents and heroic recoveries*. Farnham: Ashgate.

Russell, C. (2019). Four modes of change: To, for, with, by. *HindSight*. 28: 8–11 [online]. Available from: https://www.skybrary.aero/bookshelf/books/4508.pdf

Shorrock, S.T. (2012). Safety culture in your hands: discussion cards for understanding and improving safety culture. In: Anderson, M. (ed.). *Contemporary Ergonomics and Human Factors 2012*. London: Taylor & Francis, pp. 321–328.

Shorrock, S.T. et al. (2011). Developing a safety culture questionnaire for European air traffic management: Learning from experience. In: Anderson, M. (ed.). *Contemporary Ergonomics and Human Factors 2011*. London: Taylor & Francis, pp. 56–63.

Sørskår, L.I.K. et al. (2019). Assessing safety climate in prehospital settings: testing psychometric properties of a common structural model in a cross-sectional and prospective study. *BMC Health Services Research*. 19(1): 674.

The Health Foundation (2011). Evidence scan: Levels of harm. London: Health Foundation [online]. Available from: https://www.health.org.uk/sites/default/files/LevelsOfHarm_0.pdf

Wagenaar, W.A., Hudson, P.T.W., Reason, J.T. (1990). Cognitive failures and accidents. *Applied Cognitive Psychology*. 4: 273–294.

Waterson, P. (2014). *Patient Safety Culture: Theory, methods and application*. Farnham: Ashgate.

Westrum, R. (2004). A typology of organisational cultures. *Quality & Safety in Health Care*. 13(2): 22–27.

World Health Organization (2009). *Patient Safety Research: better knowledge for better care*. Geneva: WHO.

Index

A
AcciMaps model of incident and accident analysis 147
action slip 134
active errors 25
adult advanced life support algorithm 118
adverse event *see* patient safety incident
affordances 52, 53
ALARP *see* as low as reasonably practicable
always events 80
analytical decision making *see* choice decision making
analytical/psychological approach 160
anchoring bias 114
anthropological approach 160
as low as reasonably practicable (ALARP) 18, 152
attention 105
authority gradient 135–136
availability bias 114

B
barriers to design in
    behavioural-based safety 56–57
    good provider fallacy 58–59
    make do and mend 57–58
    normalisation of deviance 58
behavioural-based safety 56–57
behavioural marker systems 102
behavioural modification 56
belongingness needs, occupational stress 90
bias, in decision making 113–114
blaming, avoidance of 145–146

C
CAA *see* Civil Aviation Authority
Café Wall illusion 106
Calgary–Cambridge guide 76, 77
Cambridge Cockpit 17
Care Opinion 80
care team, questions to guide 152–153
change blindness 105
Chartered Institute of Ergonomics and Human Factors (CIEHF) 4
CHFG *see* Clinical Human Factors Group
choice decision making 118–119
CIEHF *see* Chartered Institute of Ergonomics and Human Factors
circadian rhythm 94
Civil Aviation Authority (CAA) 5, 110
clinical error *see* human error
Clinical Human Factors Group (CHFG) 19
    definition of human factors 3
co-design 51
    and service improvement, public involvement in 79–80
        always events 80
        feedback systems 80
cognitive human factors/ergonomics 18, 64–65
cognitive task load (CTL) model 132–133
command gradient *see* authority gradient
communication 136–138
    closed loop process 136
    and feedback to staff 122
    impaired 92
    responsibilities in 137
    tools for team situation awareness 129–130
complex care systems 33–34
    human error vs. systems thinking 36–37
    workarounds and trade-offs 35–36
    work-as-done vs. work-as-imagined 34–35
complex system 33
complicated system 32–33
comprehension, level of situation awareness 106–107
confirmation bias 114
consultation, definition of 75–76
contemporary psychology 88
contextual factors 148
creative decision making 119, 120
Crew Resource Management (CRM) 18, 102
CTL model *see* cognitive task load (CTL) model
CUS tool 138

D
decision making 103, 128–131
    advantages and pitfalls of methods 119–120
    bias 113–114
    choice 118–119
    creative 119, 120

Index

evolution of 111–112
factors influencing 120–122
impaired 92
model of 114–115
paramedic 114
recognition-primed 115–117, 119
rule-based 117–118, 119
shared 74–75
System 1 and System 2 thinking, 112–113
defibrillators 55–56
depression 86
design error 51
Design of Everyday Things, The 51
design *see* human-centred design
dialogue principles 61–62
discussion cards 164–168
Dual Process Theory 112

E
efficiency–thoroughness trade-offs 36
emergent expertise 20
emergent outcomes 147–148
emotional well-being of ambulance clinicians 144
employee health and well-being 84
Endsley's model 104–107
environment 37
environmental capture 134
esteem needs, occupational stress 90
EUROCONTROL Safety Culture Discussion Cards 164–168
eustress 85
events
  learning from *see* learning, from events
  reporting of *see* reporting of events
  reviewing *see* reviewing events
  safety and risk-related terminology 142

F
factors affecting humans 21
factors of humans 21, 101
falls referral pathway 39–41
fatigue 94–96
feedback systems 80
field study 63
1st stories 145
fundamental attribution error 57

G
good provider fallacy 58–59

H
handovers 76
health, definition of 84

heuristics 63, 113
HF/E *see* human factors/ergonomics
history of HF 15–22
  development in healthcare 18–20
history-taking 75, 76
human–automation interaction 18
human-centred design (HCD) 49–50
  barriers in healthcare
    behavioural-based safety 56–57
    good provider fallacy 58–59
    make do and mend 57–58
    normalisation of deviance 58
  definition of 61
  design focusing on people
    human-centred design 59–62
    usability 62–63
    user-centred design 59
  designing with people 51
  human factors/ergonomics
    cognitive 64–65
    organisational 66–67
    physical 63–64
  for interactive systems 61
  for patient safety 52, 54
    defibrillator case study 55–56
  role and importance of 50–51
human–computer interaction 18, 62
human error 7, 23–24
  definition of 24–25
  paramedic error, looking beyond 26
  vs. systems thinking 36–37
  types of 25–26
  views of 26–28
human factors/ergonomics (HF/E)
  aims of 2
  birth of 15–16
  definitions 3
    alternative definitions 3
    IEA definition 4
    terminology 4–5
  description of 1–3
  design domains in
    cognitive 64–65
    organisational 66–67
    physical 63–64
  development in healthcare 18–20
  evaluation methods for usability 63
  in forensics and litigation 18
  growth of 17–18
  misconceptions of 8–9
  models for application 9–10
  for patient safety 5–7
    person-centred approach 7
    Safety-I and Safety-II, 8

172

Index

systems approach 7
in practice today 20
roots of 16–17
suggested levels of input in healthcare 12
types of 20–21

I

IEA *see* International Ergonomics Association
illness-related factors, patient participation and 78
illusion 106
impaired communication 92
impaired decision making 92
impaired leadership 92
impaired performance 92
impaired situation awareness 92
inattentional blindness 105
incident reporting and learning systems 143–144
informed culture 161
International Ergonomics Association (IEA) 2, 3, 4
International Organization for Standardization (ISO) 61–62
International Paramedic Anxiety Wellbeing and Stress (IPAWS) 93
inter-task constraints 135
intuitive decision making *see* recognition-primed decision making
IPAWS *see* International Paramedic Anxiety Wellbeing and Stress
ISO *see* International Organization for Standardization

J

just culture 161

L

leadership *see also* task allocation; task management
  impaired 92
  influence on types of safety culture 161
  teamwork in paramedic practice 131–135
learning
  culture 161
  from events 141–142
    care system resilience 152–153
    never event lists, limitations of 151–152
    Safety-I and Safety-II thinking 150–151
  linear thinking and methods limitations 149–150
local rationality 148–149
long-term memory 106, 109–110
low oxygen saturations, situation awareness 108

M

'make do and mend,' 57–58
making decisions *see* decision making
Maslow's Hierarchy of Needs 89–90
medical error 19
medication packaging 27
memory in situation awareness 109–110
mental ill-health 83
mental model 103
mental well-being 83 *see also* well-being of paramedic
metacognition 113
Montgomery v NHS Lanarkshire 74
Müller-Lyer illusion 106

N

natural mapping 52, 54
naturalistic decision making 112
Neighbour's model 76
never events 141
  lists, limitations of 151–152
non-systems approach 41
non-technical skills 5, 101–102 *see also* decision making; situation awareness
  impact of stress on 90–92
non-technical skills assessment frameworks (NOTECHS) 102
non-verbal communication 136
normalisation of deviance 58
Norman door 52, 53

O

occupational stress 83, 87–89
  Maslow's Hierarchy of Needs 89–90
  non-technical skills, impact of stress on 90–92
  sources of stress 90
'onion' models 9–10
open culture 161
organisation 37
organisational human factors/ergonomics 66–67
organisational performance 122
overlapping functionality 134–135

P

PACE tool 138
paramedic decision making 114
paramedic error 26
paramedic factors, patient participation and 78–79
paramedic–patient interaction 75–76
patient
  consultation 75–76

173

Index

as an element of system 71–72
engagement for patient safety 72–73
highlighting when things go wrong
  checking patient care record 77
  handovers 76
paramedic–patient interaction 75–76
participation, factors influencing 77–78
  illness-related factors 78
  paramedic factors 78–79
  patient-related factors 78
person-centred care 73
  shared decision making 74–75
public involvement in co-design and service improvement 79–80
  always events 80
  feedback systems 80
Patient and Public Involvement (PPI) 72, 79
patient care record 77
patient-related factors, patient participation and 78
patient safety 5–7
  design for 52, 54
  incident 6
  patient engagement for 72–73
  person-centred approach 7
  Safety-I and Safety-II, 8
  systems approach 7
  systems engineering initiative for 11
Patient Safety Partner (PSP) 79
Pendleton's model 76
perception, level of situation awareness 105
perfection myth 57
person approach 56–57
person-centred care 7, 73
  shared decision making 74–75
physical human factors/ergonomics 63–64
physiological needs, occupational stress 90
pilot error 15–16
post-traumatic stress disorder (PTSD) 86
PPI see Patient and Public Involvement
pragmatic/experience-based approach 160
pre-hospital clinical care 108–109
pre-hospital system, well-being in 85–87
priming effect 114
procurement 62
'Project A,' 87
projection, level of situation awareness 107
PSP see Patient Safety Partner
PTSD see post-traumatic stress disorder
public involvement
  in co-design and service improvement 79–80
    always events 80
    feedback systems 80
punishment myth 57

R

rational model of decision making 112
recognition-primed decision making 112, 115–117, 119
reporting culture 161
reporting of events
  emotional well-being 144
  incident reporting and learning systems 143
  safety and risk-related terminology 142
resources 122
  limitations 134
retrospective systemic accident model 9
reviewing events
  blaming, avoidance of 145–146
  1st and 2nd stories 145
  linear thinking and methods limitations 149–150
  systems thinking, integration in analytical process 146–149
risk aversion 122
road traffic collision, situation awareness 108–109
rule-based decision making 117–118, 119

S

safety and security needs, occupational stress 90
safety climate
  safety culture vs., 158
  survey scores by 162–163
safety culture
  for ambulance services 160–162
  EUROCONTROL Safety Culture Discussion Cards 165–168
  importance of 158–159
  leadership influence on types of 161
  meaning of 157–158
  problem with measuring 162–163
  safety climate vs., 158
  theory into practice 164–165
  understanding 160
Safety-I thinking 8, 150–151
Safety-II thinking 8, 150–151
'SBAR' tool 137
'SBARR' tool 137
scientific management 16
2nd stories 145
second victims 144
SEIPS Model see Systems Engineering Initiative for Patient Safety (SEIPS) Model
self-actualisation 90
shared decision making 74–75
shift working 95
short-term memory 106, 109–110

174

Index

signage 60
simple system 32
situation awareness 103–104
   examples of 107–109
   factors influencing 120–122
   impaired 92
   levels of 104–105
      comprehension 106–107
      perception 105
      projection 107
   maintaining 110–111
   role of memory in 109–110
   team *see* team situation awareness
situational factors 148
socio-technical system 3, 21, 146–147
staff training and development, inadequate 121
'sterile cockpit' concept 110
STEW model *see* Systems Thinking for Everyday Work (STEW) model
stress *see also* occupational stress
   definition of 87
   sources of 90
   work system elements associated with 91
Stryker Physio Control LIFEPAK 12 and 15 cardiac monitor/defibrillators 55
survey questionnaires 162–163
Swiss Cheese model 9
SWOT analysis 168
system
   complex 33
   complicated 32–33
   definition of 31–32
   performance 85
   simple 32
   types of 32–33
System 1 thinking 112–113
System 2 thinking 113
systems approach 7
Systems Engineering Initiative for Patient Safety (SEIPS) Model 10, 37–39, 51, 73, 147
   to out-of-hospital falls pathways 39–41
systems interaction approach 92–93
systems thinking 31
   for everyday work 42
   human error vs., 36–37
   incident reporting and learning systems 143–144
   integrating in analytical process 146–147
      emergent outcomes 147–148
      local rationality 148–149
      look 'up and out' rather than 'down and in', 149
      situational and contextual issues 148

Systems Engineering Initiative for Patient Safety 37–39
   to out-of-hospital falls pathways 39–41
Systems Thinking for Everyday Work 41–42
   to pre-hospital case 42–46
Systems Thinking for Everyday Work (STEW) model 41–42, 147
   to pre-hospital case 42, 44–46
   principles for use during group discussions 43

T

target fixation 134
task allocation
   definition of 131
   vs. task management 132
task instability 134
task management
   cognitive task load model 132–133
   definition of 131
   failures in 132–133
   task allocation vs., 132
   Yerkes–Dodson model 133–135
tasks 37
team-based approach 141–142
team formation 126–127
   stages 127–128s
Team Resource Management (TRM) 5, 102
team situation awareness 128–129
   communication tools for building 129–130
   requirements 129
   response to loss of 130–131
   strata of 129
teams, definition of 126
teamwork in paramedic practice 125–126
   authority gradients 135–136
   communication 136–138
   forming teams 126–128
   scenario 125
   task management and leadership 131–135
   team situation awareness and decision making 128–131
time and motion study 16
To Err is Human 6, 8, 18, 23
tools and technologies 37
trade-offs 35–36
TRM *see* Team Resource Management
tunnel vision 105
two-challenge rule 137–138

U

usability 62–63
   testing 63
   walkthrough 63
user-centred design 59

Index

V

verbal communication 136

W

WAD *see* work-as-done
WAI *see* work-as-imagined
well-being of paramedic 83–84
   fatigue 94–96
   occupational stress 87–89
      Maslow's Hierarchy of Needs 89–90
      non-technical skills, impact of stress on 90–92
      sources of stress 90
   in pre-hospital system 85–87
   systems approaches to managing stress and 92–94
   in workplace 84–87
   work processes and system performance 85
workarounds 35–36
work-as-done (WAD) 59
   vs. work-as-imagined 34–35
work-as-imagined (WAI) 59
   work-as-done vs., 34–35
working memory 106, 109
workplace well-being
   in pre-hospital system 85–87
   work processes and system performance 85
work processes 85
World Health Organization (WHO) 19, 84

Y

Yerkes–Dodson model 133

Other Titles of Interest

Decision Making in Paramedic Practice
By Andy Collen
ISBN: 9781859596418

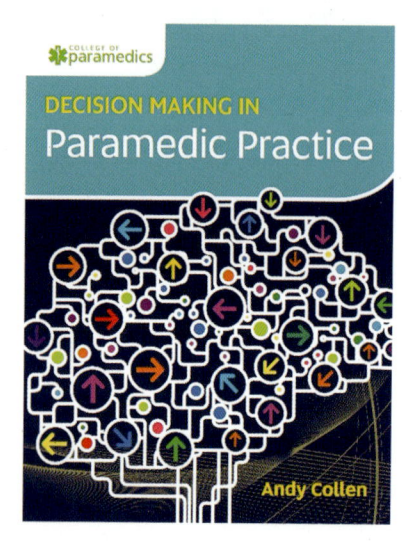

Law and Ethics for Paramedics
Edited by Georgette Eaton
ISBN: 9781859596678

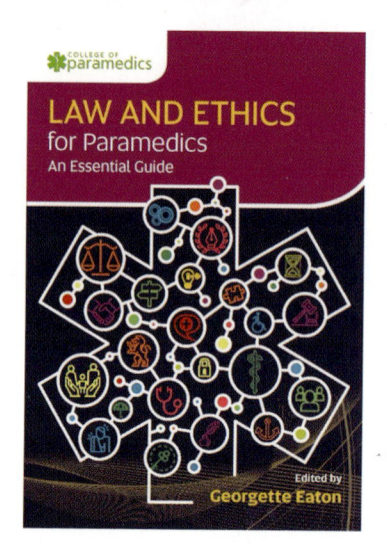

Independent Prescribing for Paramedics
By Amanda Blaber, Hannah Morris and Andy Collen
ISBN: 9781859597873

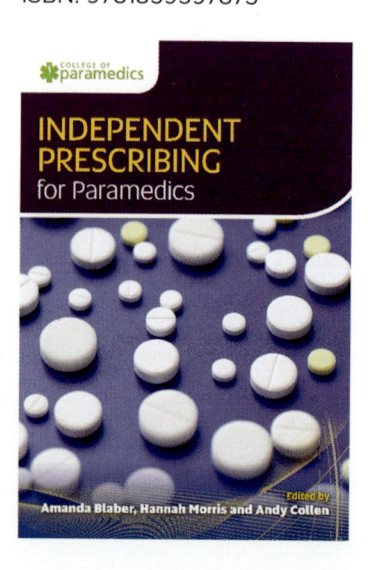

Palliative and End of Life Care for Paramedics
Edited by Tania Blackmore
ISBN: 9781859596715

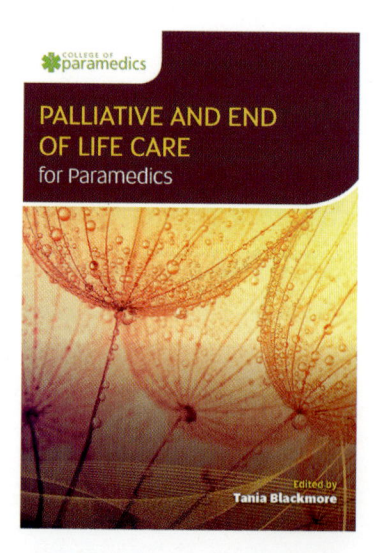